Artificial Intelligence for Accurate Analysis and Detection of Autism Spectrum Disorder

Sandeep Kautish
Lord Buddha Education Foundation, Nepal & Asia Pacific University of Technology & Innovation, Malaysia

Gaurav Dhiman
Government Bikram College of Commerce, India

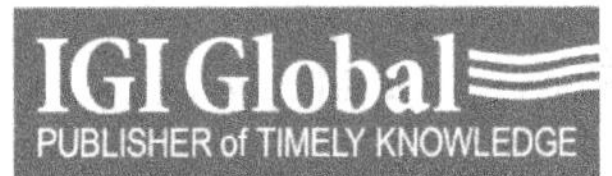

A volume in the Advances in Medical Diagnosis, Treatment, and Care (AMDTC) Book Series

Published in the United States of America by
IGI Global
Medical Information Science Reference (an imprint of IGI Global)
701 E. Chocolate Avenue
Hershey PA, USA 17033
Tel: 717-533-8845
Fax: 717-533-8661
E-mail: cust@igi-global.com
Web site: http://www.igi-global.com

Library of Congress Cataloging-in-Publication Data

Names: Kautish, Sandeep Kumar, 1981- editor. | Dhiman, Gaurav, 1993- editor.
Title: Artificial intelligence for accurate analysis and detection of autism spectrum disorder / Sandeep Kautish and Gaurav Dhiman, editor.
Description: Hershey, PA : Medical Information Science Reference, [2021] | Includes bibliographical references and index. | Summary: "This book includes accumulated recent research and advances in the field of Autism spectrum disorder early detection and diagnosis enabled by Artificial Intelligence (AI) techniques i.e. apps and therapies"-- Provided by publisher.
Identifiers: LCCN 2021027452 (print) | LCCN 2021027453 (ebook) | ISBN 9781799874607 (h/c) | ISBN 9781799874614 (s/c) | ISBN 9781799874621 (eISBN)
Subjects: MESH: Autism Spectrum Disorder--diagnosis | Artificial Intelligence | Early Diagnosis | Autism Spectrum Disorder--therapy
Classification: LCC RC553.A88 (print) | LCC RC553.A88 (ebook) | NLM WS 350.8.P4 | DDC 616.85/88200285--dc23
LC record available at https://lccn.loc.gov/2021027452
LC ebook record available at https://lccn.loc.gov/2021027453

This book is published in the IGI Global book series Advances in Medical Diagnosis, Treatment, and Care (AMDTC) (ISSN: 2475-6628; eISSN: 2475-6636)

British Cataloguing in Publication Data
A Cataloguing in Publication record for this book is available from the British Library.

All work contributed to this book is new, previously-unpublished material.
The views expressed in this book are those of the authors, but not necessarily of the publisher.

For electronic access to this publication, please contact: eresources@igi-global.com.

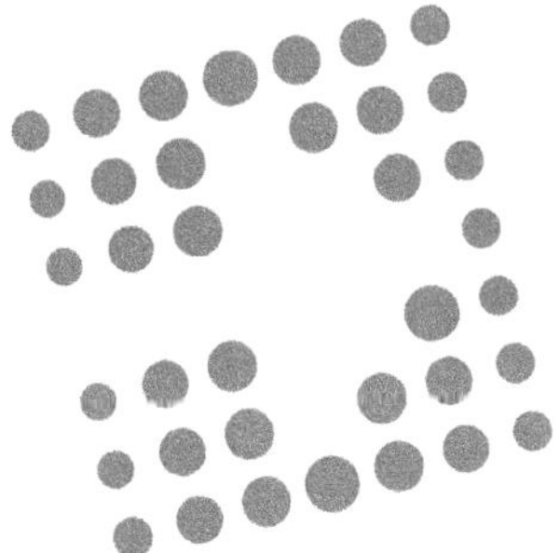

Advances in Medical Diagnosis, Treatment, and Care (AMDTC) Book Series

ISSN:2475-6628
EISSN:2475-6636

MISSION

Advancements in medicine have prolonged the life expectancy of individuals all over the world. Once life-threatening conditions have become significantly easier to treat and even cure in many cases. Continued research in the medical field will further improve the quality of life, longevity, and wellbeing of individuals.

The **Advances in Medical Diagnosis, Treatment, and Care (AMDTC)** book series seeks to highlight publications on innovative treatment methodologies, diagnosis tools and techniques, and best practices for patient care. Comprised of comprehensive resources aimed to assist professionals in the medical field apply the latest innovations in the identification and management of medical conditions as well as patient care and interaction, the books within the AMDTC series are relevant to the research and practical needs of medical practitioners, researchers, students, and hospital administrators.

COVERAGE

- Diagnostic Medicine
- Critical Care
- Disease Management
- Internal Medicine
- Alternative Medicine
- Experimental Medicine
- Emergency Medicine
- Disease Prevention
- Medical Testing
- Cancer Treatment

IGI Global is currently accepting manuscripts for publication within this series. To submit a proposal for a volume in this series, please contact our Acquisition Editors at Acquisitions@igi-global.com or visit: http://www.igi-global.com/publish/.

The Advances in Medical Diagnosis, Treatment, and Care (AMDTC) Book Series (ISSN 2475-6628) is published by IGI Global, 701 E. Chocolate Avenue, Hershey, PA 17033-1240, USA, www.igi-global.com. This series is composed of titles available for purchase individually; each title is edited to be contextually exclusive from any other title within the series. For pricing and ordering information please visit http://www.igi-global.com/book-series/advances-medical-diagnosis-treatment-care/129618. Postmaster: Send all address changes to above address.

Titles in this Series

For a list of additional titles in this series, please visit:
http://www.igi-global.com/book-series/advances-medical-diagnosis-treatment-care/129618

Strategies to Overcome Superbug Invasions Emerging Research and Opportunities
Dimple Sethi Chopra (Punjabi University, India) and Ankur Kaul (Institute of Nuclear Medicine and Allied Sciences, India)
Medical Information Science Reference • © 2021 • 319pp • H/C (ISBN: 9781799803072) • US $225.00

Integrated Care and Fall Prevention in Active and Healthy Aging
Patrik Eklund (Umea University, Sweden)
Medical Information Science Reference • © 2021 • 335pp • H/C (ISBN: 9781799844112) • US $345.00

Cases on Applied and Therapeutic Humor
Michael K. Cundall Jr. (North Carolina A&T State University, USA) and Stephanie Kelly (North Carolina A&T State University, USA)
Medical Information Science Reference • © 2021 • 267pp • H/C (ISBN: 9781799845287) • US $255.00

Diagnostic and Treatment Methods for Ulcerative Colitis and Colitis-Associated Cancer
Ashok Kumar Pandurangan (B. S. Abdur Rahman Crescent Institute of Science and Technology, India)
Medical Information Science Reference • © 2021 • 309pp • H/C (ISBN: 9781799835806) • US $295.00

Enhancing the Therapeutic Efficacy of Herbal Formulations
Rajesh Kumar Kesharwani (Nehru Gram Bharati (Deemed), Prayagraj, India) Raj K. Keservani (Faculty of B. Pharmacy, CSM Group of Institutions, Prayagraj, India) and Anil K. Sharma (GD Goenka University, India)
Medical Information Science Reference • © 2021 • 367pp • H/C (ISBN: 9781799844532) • US $265.00

Climate Change and Its Impact on Fertility
Khursheed Ahmad Wani (Goverment Degree College, Bijbehara, India) and Nibedita Naha (ICMR, National Institute of Occupational Health, Ahmedabad, India)
Medical Information Science Reference • © 2021 • 416pp • H/C (ISBN: 9781799844808) • US $265.00

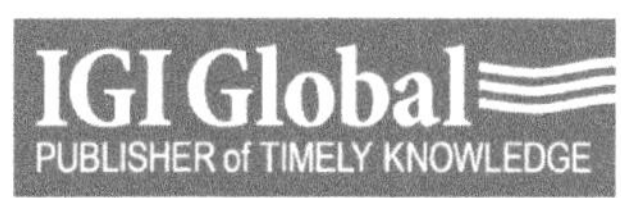

701 East Chocolate Avenue, Hershey, PA 17033, USA
Tel: 717-533-8845 x100 • Fax: 717-533-8661
E-Mail: cust@igi-global.com • www.igi-global.com

Editorial Advisory Board

Table of Contents

Detailed Table of Contents

Autism spectrum disorder (ASD) is one of the most common diseases that cause difficulties for an individual to express his/her emotions or to understand other's emotions. ASD has become a challenging problem as its symptoms are unpredictable. The main symptoms of ASD include problems such as abnormal social reciprocity, nonverbal communication, sensory abnormalities, etc. To understand such abnormalities, there is a requirement of some learning tools. It has been witnessed that facial expression images, eye tracking, and neuroimage have been shown as effective tools for analysis of abnormalities that had occurred in both grey and white matter of the brain. Many researchers focused their work on the classification problem of ASD disorder from healthy subjects but still didn't reach effective diagnosis and healing tools. As with the advancement of digital image processing, it has become feasible to use these technologies for accurate diagnosis of ASD subjects. These technologies are integrated with deep learning for the identification and treatment of ASD.

The major purpose of these research works has been for the rapid, reliable diagnosis of autism disorder by a new neuro-fuzzy autism identification technique. The highly affected region for each person is highlighted by this procedure. This research, which involves autism and regular group, included two classes of adolescents. This neuro-fuzzy method was developed by the experts using fuzzy-logical principles. The two classes were checked on the system. The developed method has been confirmed to distinguish easily between autistic participants and normal participants with increased precision. The engineered device has also been found to be 97.3% precise and 98.9% specific. The engineered instrument can be used by physicians to diagnose autism in conjunction with the seriousness of autism and to precisely and immediately illuminate the highly affected region.

Over the last few years, academic institutions have conducted a number of programmes to help school boards, colleges, and schools of autism spectrum educating pupils (ASD). Autism spectrum disorder (ASD) is a complicated neurological disorder which affects many skills over a lifetime. The main aim of the chapter is to examine the topic of autism and identify autism levels with furious logic classification algorithms using the artificial neural network. Data mining has generally been recognized as a method of decision making to promote higher use of resources for autism students.

Autism spectrum disorder (ASD) is an ongoing neurodevelopmental disorder, with repeated behavior called stereotypical movement autism (SMM). Some recent experiments with accelerometer features as feedback to computer classifiers demonstrate positive findings in persons with autistic motor disorders for the automobile detection of stereotypical motor motions (SMM). To date, several methods for detecting and recognizing SMMs have been introduced. In this context, the authors suggest an approach of deep learning for recognition of SMM, namely deep convolution neural networks (DCNN). They also implemented a robust DCNN model for the identification of SMM in order to solve stereotypical motor movements (SMM), which thus outperform state-of-the-art SMM classification work.

Autism spectrum disorder (ASD) is a neuro disorder in which a person's contact and connection with others has a lifetime impact. In all levels of development, autism can be diagnosed as a "behavioural condition," since signs generally occur within the first two years of life. The ASD problem begins with puberty and goes on in adolescence and adulthood. In this chapter, an effort is being made to use the supporting vector machine (SVM) and the convolutionary neural network (CNN) for prediction and interpretation of children's ASD problems based on the increased use of machine learning methodology in the research dimension of medical diagnostics. On freely accessible autistic spectrum disorder screening dates in children's datasets, the suggested approaches are tested. Using different techniques of machine learning, the findings clearly conclude that CNN-based prediction models perform more precisely on the dataset for autistic spectrum disorders.

Autism spectrum disorder (ASD) is growing faster than ever before. Autism detection is costly and time intensive with screening procedures. Autism can be detected at an early stage by the development of artificial intelligence and machine learning (ML). While a number of experiments using many approaches were conducted, these studies provided no conclusion as to the prediction of autism characteristics in various age groups. This chapter is therefore intended to suggest an accurate MLASD predictive model based on the ML methodology to prevent ASD for people of all ages. It is a method for prediction. This survey was conducted to develop and

Preface

Autism Spectrum Disorder (ASD) is a known as a kind of neuro-disorder in which a person may face problems in interaction and communication with others and it may continue for lifetime. As per medical experts, Autism Disorder can be diagnosed at any stage. It is also being referred as a "behavioral disease" because, in general, the symptoms appear in the first two years. Everyday social interactions with family members and other persons of the ASD affected children can become challenging. Autism spectrum disorder (ASD) appears to have a vivid increase over the last couple of years. Recent reports reveals that the prevalence of autism spectrum disorder (ASD) among children is continuously increasing (as of 2017, in Japan 161 children per 10,000 children, in UK 94 children per 10,000 children, in USA 66 children per 10,000 children). Actually, despite considerable progress in understanding the neurobiology of ASD, established treatments for core symptoms are still not available. It is crucial to provide researchers and clinicians with the most updated information on the clinical features, etiopathogenesis and therapeutic strategies for the patients as well as to shed light on the other psychiatric conditions often associated with ASD.

Our book will be one of very first efforts to accumulate recent researches and advances in the field of Autism spectrum disorder early detection and diagnosis enabled by Artificial Intelligence (AI) techniques i.e. apps and therapies. Recent studies reveal that AI enabled technologies and techniques i.e. medical robots can help children with ASD to develop the social skills which can enable them to communicate effectively. Such techniques will not only help them to improve their communication skills but also social and emotional skills as well. AI can also help in early diagnosis of ASD which is extremely important as late diagnosis may delay in getting therapies and services that should be available at very early stage. AI-aided diagnosis i.e. Deep Learning and Machine Learning algorithms are efficient in the way to confirm of a diagnosis or suggest the need for further evaluation.

The book will serve following purposes:

- To showcase the recent innovations, trends, and concerns as well as applied challenges encountered and solutions adopted in the field of AI enabled diagnosis, screening and analysis of Autism Spectrum Disorder
- To provide an excellent reference material for academic scientists, researcher and research scholars active in the research areas of Autism Spectrum Disorder
- The proposed book will empower the rethinking processes i.e. how we integrate information, analyze data, and use the resulting perceptions to advance decision making process in Autism Spectrum Disorder
- This book will lay down theoretical aspects, framework, system architecture implementation, validation, tools and techniques in relation to uses of AI in Autism Spectrum Disorder

Chapter 1 is mainly focused on the exploration of machine learning or deep learning applications for ASD diagnosis. The chapter gives a brief description of the result analysis of existing techniques that concludes with the efficiency of the CNN model for ASD diagnosis. Thus, the proposed methodology uses the computer vision application and CNN model for diagnosis of ASD efficiently. The study also gives future research direction to use the advancement of digital image processing to develop a more feasible framework for accurate diagnosis of ASD subjects with the integration of deep learning.

Chapter 2 has a major purpose for the rapid, reliable diagnosis of autism disorder by a new neuro-fuzzy autism identification technique. The two classes were checked on the system. The chapter discusses autism and the many manifestations of autism and compares the efficiency of popular informatics with the fleeting thinking of the neuro-fuzzy method. The results of this analysis suggest that the psychometric properties of the neuro-fuzzy mechanism are strong. The method for evaluating autism is accurate and true.

Chapter 3 examines the topic of autism, and identifies autism levels with furious logic classification algorithms using the Artificial Neural Network. Autism spectrum disorders (ASDs) are determined in the presence of restricted attention and repeated conduct, by deficiency of social functioning and expression. The present work refers to the issue of autism and contrasts the efficiency of popular computer education techniques with the fugitive reasoning of the Artificial Neural Network. The findings support the development potential of a successful SIB surveillance scheme, which is one of the most dangerous issues in ASD.

Chapter 4 suggests an approach of deep learning for recognition of Stereotypical Motor Motions (SMM), namely, deep convolution neural networks (DCNN). Theoretical studies have shown that the DCNN approaches the conventional handcrafted definition of the deeper neural network. This discovery confirms initial hypothesis that deep neural networks can train and move more reliable SMM sensing systems. The study shows the feasibility of embedded functionality learning. This work is an early attempt to improve SMM detectors in real time. A device can be built into a smartphone application for the omnipresent identification of SMM.

Chapter 5 narrates that Autism can be diagnosed as a behavioural condition, since signs generally occur within the first two years of life. The problem begins with puberty and goes on in adolescence and adulthood. In this paper, two machine learning approaches have been used for the diagnosis of Autism Spectrum Disorder (ASD). Diverse criteria have been used for success assessment in nonclinical data set analysis of ASD detection models. The CNN classifier has reached a high degree of precision and the results show that an autism-spectrum condition CNN model should be used instead of a conventional machine learning classification.

Chapter 6 explains that Autism can be expected at an early stage by the development of artificial intelligence and machine learning (ML). This paper is therefore intended to suggest an accurate MLASD predictive model based on the ML methodology to prevent ASD for people of all ages. AQ-10 data collection was used to test the proposed pattern. The findings of the evaluation reveal that the proposed prediction model has improved results in terms of consistency, specificity, sensitivity and dataset accuracy. Autism with 96.06%, 97.78%, and 93.54% for children, teenagers and adults, can be predicted by the proposed model, by using the AQ-10 dataset.

Chapter 7 discusses about Learning disabilities which are different type of neurologically based processing problems. Children face many difficulties such as writing, reading and mathematics. Dyslexia is most common type of learning disability. Children having dyslexia problems in language processing, decode the words, identifying the sound of letters and reading fluently. The most techniques are available in Arabic, Malay, English but not for Punjabi spoken dyslexic children. Lacks of assistive technologies are barriers for dyslexics in their learning. The chapter is focusing on available assistive techniques and developing an ASR application based on machine learning in Punjabi regional language. This technique will be very helpful for Punjabi spoken dyslexic children in their learning skills.

Chapter 8 discusses Artificial Intelligence which can be termed as a powerful tool that has the capability to process huge sums of information with ease and assess patterns created over a period of time to give significant results or suggestions. In this book chapter, is discussed about ASD, current role of AI in advancing autistic lives including detection, analysis and treatment of ASD. The chapter examines current and provides support for the future advancements, including the idea of the use of "Mouse-less Cursor Control" and "Brain- Computer Interface" based developments, for improving social abilities and reducing the communication & motor difficulties faced by people with ASD. The discussed utilities are already being used by many people including people dealing with Quadriplegia, Arthritis and more, but not much by autistic people. Hence, an attempt is made to highlight the lesser-explored technologies which can be exploited to add convenience to the autistic lives in manifold ways.

In Chapter 9, the authors presented several Machine Learning (ML) models based on Support Vector Machines (SVM), Naïve Bayes (NB), k-Nearest Neighbours (KNN) and Decision Trees (DT) algorithms to diagnose the autism in the individuals. The authors also improved the performance of the ML models with the help of optimal subset of features selected using various well-known evolutionary optimization algorithms like GA and BTLBO. The experimental setup and discussion of results on various ASD datasets (children, adolescent and adult) of UCI repository are specified in this chapter.

Acknowledgment

This book is my third book with IGI Global, and I am delighted to complete this during this pandemic era. I congratulate all chapter authors for their valuable submissions and keeping patience during critical review process. I wish to thank all reviewers as well who spared their precious time for the review process.

I am thankful to my co-editor Dr Gaurav Dhiman for his valuable contribution. Also I thank my wife, Yogita and son, Devansh and my parents for giving me eternal happiness and support for the entire process.

Last but not the least, I am thankful to almighty god for blessing me with wonderful life and showing me right paths in my all ups and downs during the so far journey of life.

Sandeep Kautish
Lord Buddha Education Foundation, Nepal and Asia Pacific University of Technology & Innovation, Malaysia

Chapter 1
Application of Image Processing for Autism Spectrum Disorder

Pradeep Bedi
Lingayas Vidyapeeth, India

S. B. Goyal
https://orcid.org/0000-0002-8411-7630
City University, Malaysia

Jugnesh Kumar
St. Andrews Institute of Technology and Management, India

Shailesh Kumar
BlueCrest College, Freetown, Sierra Leone

ABSTRACT

Autism spectrum disorder (ASD) is one of the most common diseases that cause difficulties for an individual to express his/her emotions or to understand other's emotions. ASD has become a challenging problem as its symptoms are unpredictable. The main symptoms of ASD include problems such as abnormal social reciprocity, nonverbal communication, sensory abnormalities, etc. To understand such abnormalities, there is a requirement of some learning tools. It has been witnessed that facial expression images, eye tracking, and neuroimage have been shown as effective tools for analysis of abnormalities that had occurred in both grey and white matter of the brain. Many researchers focused their work on the classification problem of ASD disorder from healthy subjects but still didn't reach effective diagnosis and healing tools. As with the advancement of digital image processing, it has become feasible to use these technologies for accurate diagnosis of ASD subjects. These technologies are integrated with deep learning for the identification and treatment of ASD.

DOI: 10.4018/978-1-7998-7460-7.ch001

1. INTRODUCTION

Autism can be categorized as the disorder of neurodevelopmental disorder which has symptoms like an early stage of shortcoming in social communication while interacting with people, being restricted and confined, and having a behavior of repetitive pattern. In the age group of fewer than five years, the main reason disabilities of mental disorders are autism. If the childhood disorders like; Attention Deficit Hyperactivity Disorder, as well as Conduct Disorder, is compared with autism then the effect of autism is for a lifetime. The symptoms of ASD can be recognized at its early stage but there are still some disabilities and pattern of behaviors are difficult to recognize as symptoms till the life of a child is affected at a significant level. Individuals with ASD would have varied limited functions or symptoms and it may differ over the period. One of the main symptoms of ASD is delayed or misinterpretation in language acquisition. It is reported that around 50 percent of people suffering from autism are incapable of framing a clear speech. ASD's one of the basic symptoms is impairment in social communication. It can be observed when the babies or young children do not respond properly to physical contact or interaction. Along with these symptoms; some other patterns like repetitive behavior or having a repetitive interest or some unusual interest in useless engrossment or some wired interest can be listed as the indicators of ASD (Kumar et al., 2019). Mostly ASD symptoms can be spotted in a child up to the age of 18 months. But many times, ASD is not diagnosed accurately in case the child is suffering limited delayed speech and such cases are diagnosed when children face problems in interacting with friends (Chen et al., 2019). Various tools, as well as approaches to do the diagnosis of ASD, are applied by doctors in conjunction with diagnostic tools. Doctors use classification methods for these types of studies (Jiang et al., 2019). In short, it can be said that machine learning algorithms are being used widely for the diagnosis of ASD.

1.1 Motivation and Scope

The term "autism spectrum disorder" refers to a group of neurodevelopmental disorders. ASD is characterized by poor emotional control and social interactions, as well as restricted interest, repetitive behaviors, and sensory hypo-/hyperreactivity. Learning, development, control, and interaction, as well as some everyday life abilities, are frequently impaired in people with an autism spectrum disorder. ASD places a significant financial strain on patients' families and society. Establishing an early and reliable diagnosis framework to distinguish ASD patients from usual controls is critical (TC). Neuroimaging techniques that have not recently been invasive and in vivo have become an area for intensive research on ASD auxiliary diagnoses. Neuroimaging technology is now widely employed in the investigation of a variety of brain illnesses, including ASD. Magnetic resonance imaging (MRI) provides high-grade three-dimensional (3D) images and detailed structural information on brain structures. The associated disorders have been subjected to morphological analyses based on MRI imaging, with promising outcomes. Therefore this chapter explores the application of image processing in the diagnosis of ASD.

1.2 Objectives

It is quite difficult to differentiate and recognize the person suffering from ASD and typical controls (TC) persons. In existing or conventional approaches, ASD/TC can be differentiated based on morphological features. So, this chapter is mainly designed to explore the benefits of image processing and deep learning to study extracted patterns of the brain from MRI or fMRI images. In this chapter, a model is also presented with features of CNN learning to perform ASD/TC classification.

1.3 Problems Statement

The main symptoms of ASD include problems such as abnormal social reciprocity, nonverbal communication, sensory abnormalities, etc. To understand such abnormalities there is the requirement of some learning tools. Many researchers focused their work on classification problem ASD disorder from healthy subjects but still didn't reached effective diagnosis and healing tool. The existing ASD diagnosis tools are mostly based on behavior observation and symptoms which can be sometimes misdiagnosed. So, to develop a more qualitative diagnosis, there is a need for advanced tools (Reyana, & Kautish, 2021, (Rani, & Kautish, 2018) and artificial intelligence interface to visualize and analyze the biological abnormalities for ASD disorders

1.4 Key Contributions

With the advancement of brain imaging with machine learning or deep learning, neuroscience has paved the way for a better understanding of the functional and structural behavior of the human brain. In traditional approaches, multiple univariant features are needed to be analyzed to find any learning pattern of the brain. Therefore, to study different brain disorders, different regions of the brain are analyzed. Whereas, deep learning (DL) or machine learning (ML) algorithms (Sampathkumar et al 2020) usually find the relationship among different sections of the brain and their feature vectors. Thus deep learning or machine learning algorithms (Kaur & Kautish, 2019) show supremacy over other existing conventional methods. Similarly, in this paper, proficiency of DL is presented here to analyze the brain structural and functional differences among ASD brain or normal brain on neuroimaging data. These advances will leads towards the improvement and diagnosis of human brain disorders more accurately.

This chapter contributes the following features:

- This chapter first of all gives an overview about autism spectrum disorder its symptoms and causes.
- This chapter then presents the application of AI for diagnosis of ASD in children and different research contributions in this field.
- This chapter further presents the application of deep learning on neurological images for ASD diagnosis.
- This chapter also proposed a framework for ASD diagnosis with the application of deep learning and image processing.
- In last, a theoretical state-of-art is presented with some existing works that can find a path for future research area.

Section 2 of this chapter gives an brief description about autism spectrum disorder along with that symptoms and causes. Section 3 and section 4 of the chapter gives a brief overview about a wide contribution of researchers for application of machine learning or artificial intelligence for ASD diagnosis. Section 5 contributes researchers' efforts for ASD diagnosis using brain neuroimaging. After observing the issues faced during the diagnosis process of ASD, section 6 proposes an architecture on brain neuroimaging for ASD diagnosis. Finally, in section 7, the conclusion and future research scope are discussed.

2. OVERVIEW OF AUTISM SPECTRUM DISORDER

Autism spectrum disorder has been detected as one of the disorders associated with brain development which does the diagnosis of a person's perceiving and socializing approach with others which can create challenges in social interaction as well as communication. This disorder includes limited patterns and some repetitive behavior patterns. In autism spectrum disorder term "spectrum" implicates a vast extent of signs and their seriousness. Autism spectrum disorder involves the traits that were determined to be different behavior childhood disintegrative disorder, Asperger's syndrome, autism, and an unspecified form of pervasive developmental disorder. "Asperger's syndrome", is the term is still used by some people or doctors for the mild end of autism spectrum disorder (Wang et al., 2018). Autism spectrum disorder starts in infancy so it creates complications while connecting to the surrounding; like in being social and interactive at school or play, like children explicit symptoms

Figure 1. Symptoms and causes of ASD

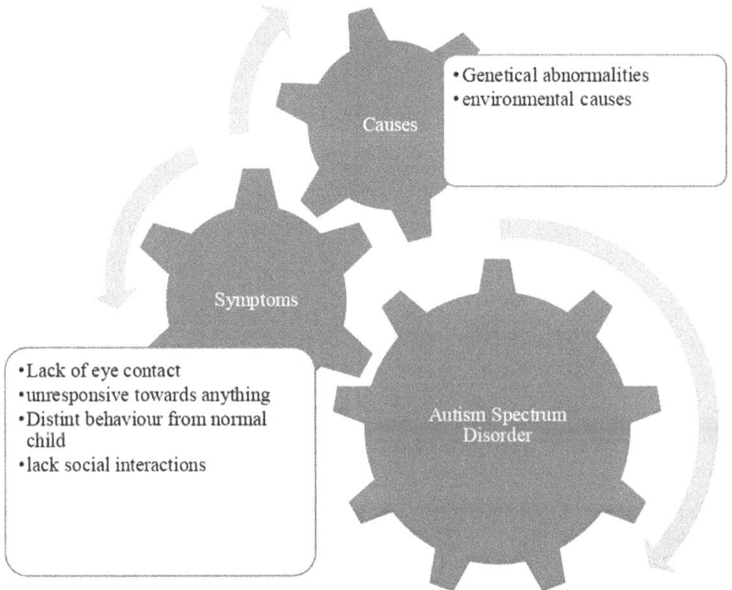

of autism during their first year. In the first year of their childhood, they develop generally and it is between the ages of 18 to 24 months when they show the symptoms of autism. Because it has no treatment of autism spectrum disorder at its severe stage so it is required to be treated at the earliest age for the betterment of the lives of many children. Fig.1. represents some symptoms and causes that needed to be focused on while the diagnosis process.

2.1 Symptoms

- The symptoms of autism spectrum disorder are expressed by some children in their early ages, like lacked eye contact, unresponsive to their name, or unresponsive to parents or family members. For the early months or years of their life, some children behave to withdraw or they may become wild or they may not develop language or lose acquired language skills. These signs are generally visible by age 2 years.
- The individual child tends to develop a distinct behavior pattern as well as seriousness level when suffering from an autism spectrum disorder. It may vary from intellectual disability to learning disability.
- Another symptom of autism spectrum disorder is that some children experience the problem of learning or few experiences lower intelligence than normal

intelligence opposite to this some other children have intelligence normal to high intelligence mean they grasp fast, then also they face in communication and the application of their knowledge in their life and to adjust with the situation of society.

- It becomes too difficult to diagnose this disorder because of the variance and severity of symptoms in each child. Determination of this disorder relies on the scale of impairments and its effect on their function ability.
- Some common signs of this disorder as explicated by some child who suffers from autism spectrum disorder are here.

2.2 Social Communication and Interaction

Autism spectrum disorders in a child and adult experience the problems in social interaction as well as in communication skills; will include any of the given signs:

- The patient remains unresponsive to their names and sometimes not even hears you.
- They dislike cuddling and holding. They like to play alone, lost in their world.
- They resist eye contact as well as they don't express through facial expression.
- They speak less or language acquisition is delayed. Sometimes they forget the learned ability to speak.
- They hesitate to start a talk or can't continue talking.
- They speak in an unusual tone or abnormal rhythm. Sometimes they talk like singsong or robot-like speech
- They try to repeat word to word, which means they do verbatim, they don't have any idea regarding its use while talking.
- They fail to comprehend easy questions or even directions.
- They fail to express their emotions and seem ignorant of the feelings of others.
- They don't express their interest.
- Their approaches for social interaction are very improper means they remain passive or aggressive or disruptive
- They face problem in recognizing nonverbal communication like they fail to interpret facial expressions of others, others body postures as well as voice tone.

2.3 Causes

There is no known cause of Autism spectrum disorder. This disorder can be either genetic or environmental and its complexity or severity may vary in all individual children (Zheng et al., 2016).

2.3.1 Environmental

The contribution of the environment is remarkable for gathering evidence supporting the pathophysiology of ASD. Exposure to the environment can greatly affect the development of the brain and it can also activate neurological processes like synaptogenesis, cell differentiation, and axon myelination. Like, according to some reports the lifestyle of maternal as well as diet can be beneficial for the brain development of the fetus. Especially, the deficiency of some important nutrients along with fatty acids is linked with neurodevelopmental results which may increase the risk of ASD. According to different studies, during pregnancy, the consumption of alcohol or recreational drugs or smoking of tobacco can be causative for structural brain anomalies like the traits of children who have ASD. The use of antidepressant medicine in the duration of pregnancy can also perturb the brain development of the fetus and can increase the risk of ASD. Other factors that are influential during pregnancy for the predisposition to ASD are inhaling air pollutants, nutritional disorder, and infection to the mother, bad economic condition as well as less education. According to a recent report, deficiency of vitamin D can lead to morphological and functional changes to the brain of children which are the typical symptoms of ASD and it also stresses the role of regular balanced nutrition to prevent the increase in symptoms of the disorder. The environmental factor that contributes to increasing the symptoms of ASD has proved to be an important research area that has been vastly studied in past years. Many studies show the connection between the environment and ASD, and to influence the predisposition to ASD not only one factor of the environment is solely but actually, it is an amalgamation of various environmental factors that are responsible. Understanding the factors of the environment which are mainly responsible for the predisposition to such neurodevelopmental disorders needs to be studied deeply and provide exact knowledge of the significant possibilities of levied with ASD so that it can provide proper guidance to guardians and doctors in taking decisions.

2.3.2 Genetics

ASD comes under an illness that is heritable that can lead to complicated cognitive changes which increases the chances of impairments while having social interaction as well as language learning. This neurodevelopmental disease has a complex genetic architecture according to the demonstration of whole-exome sequencing (WES), cytogenetics, and association studies. The clear contribution heritable factors to ASD, are shown by twin and family studies. The main diseases linked to ASD are fragile X syndrome (FXS) and tuberous sclerosis (TS). They have pathophysiological mechanisms that are quite the same as those detected in ASD sufferers, who have abnormal mRNA translation and increased protein synthesis.

3. APPLICATION OF AI FOR CHILDREN WITH ASD

Autism is a lifelong condition that affects how an individual communicates and reacts with people around him. ASD is a type of disability that shows social interaction, speech, and behavior issues. One initiative is to associate children with the NAO robot artificial intelligence (AI).

Many recent attempts on the robotic observation and contact platform have been carried out. AI robots have been shown to encourage children to look for a long time. If an autistic person interacted with an AI robot, the timespan was increased between them; children began to speak to the AI robot and were able to achieve higher scores with certain types of speech behavior appraisal. For children with ASD, it is easy and fun to communicate and read with a simple humanoid AI robot when compared with the nuanced expressions of their faces and their bodies (Coco et al., 2018). An AI robot is a most common Research Robot and a very attractive, attractive, and customized robot partner.

After learning and practicing, the AI robots will communicate with humans and document all interactions. Photo books are a genre of books with clearer pictures and fewer words that are more readable and understandable. Many children with ASD's abilities, including reading, expressing and understanding, role reversal, and expression of feelings, also improve successfully. Most image books for children are also used to optimize dialogue sharing to have a greater communication impact. Picture books are one category of books that are independent and can present plots, knowledge, beliefs, etc with plain, straightforward pictures and characters. Most scholars believe that photo books help children grow up and cultivate the separate intelligence of the moral universe profoundly. These facts present the possibility and difficulty of combining AI robots and childhood photo books, with the goal that the AI robot can automatically inform autistic children of many relevant pictorial books in conjunction with their content (Swanson et al., 2018).

The research increase in humanoid robots is evidence of a paradigm shift from independent research towards socially supportive robotics and human-friendly robots. Any of the latest literature findings suggest that ASD children are intrigued with electronic components, equipment, and robots. The AI robot was designed to look open and present emotions like a person. It is one of the world's most popular AI robots. The overall look of the AI robot is seen by 3. Some robotics in recovery therapy are currently being introduced and the AI robot is now extensively used in medical science. Children with ASD should learn how to understand human feelings and perceive their routine and repeated behavior. A variety of topic research is done and the results indicate that children with ASD show greater emotional experiences in interacting with the AI Robot than with a human counterpart by merely conversing and behaving and several different kinds of coping techniques for disease remission are invented. In a series of four-person subject tests for motor imitation, it became known that when they associate with an imitative robot, children with ASD show more social behaviors than a human partner. Furthermore, children with ASD earned better ratings on stereotyped actions as well as communication tests compared with their normal class in the AI robot-based intervention class. Furthermore, children with ASD appear to be more mindful of inanimate objects than nonverbal social cues and prefer the AI robot sound to a real human when starting communication. The AI robot can also support friends with a kid with autism. Moreover, several researchers aim to sharpen the software context to improve communication strategies between ASD children and the AI robot. To create a better communication environment for robotics, in addition to the robotic visual system, the system uses external cameras to adopt new procedures in the field of Human Robotic Interaction (HRI) based on ASD therapy and in particular for non-technical experts to take part in robotic surgeries during the treatment. However, the contact study between the kid and the AI robot is very small (or no) in the form of chats and readings. For children with ASD, reading and communicating are more complex than ordinary children, but they do have literacy requirements. Their desire to communicate can be influenced by reading the books they are involved in. Their commitment and progress in school can have a positive impact. Children with ASD are believed to have to read more and to be much more profitable by reading appropriate picture books

Coco et al., (2018) introduced a technological structure efficient to unite various visual cues for capturing the behavioral trend with an ASD treatment. It is an analytical pipeline involving detection of a face gaze calculation, landmark extraction, identification of facial expression, and pose of head estimation based and has been useful for detecting behavioral characteristics at the time of interaction among multiple children, ASD affected, and a humanoid robot.

Imitation skill learning is supposed as a core deficiency area for children with ASD and Swanson et al. (2018) offered a novel robot-mediated intervention system for it. The Robot-mediated Imitation Skill Training Architecture (RISTA) is planned in such a manner to prevail either entirely autonomously or in communion with a human therapist depending on the requirement of intervention. Initial outcomes represent that this novel robotic system is more attentive than the children with ASD and instructs gestures more efficiently than a human therapist.

Zheng et al. (2016) offered a novel corporative virtual environment (CVE)-dependent social platform for ASD interference. The advancement of CVE technology for ASD interference is helpful in the building of a novel inferior-cost environment for interference that will support the collaboration with peers and give communication flexibility. In the current Communication-advancement CVE system, two children can play the interactive games in a series in the environment of virtual reality with the help of common gestures of hand to move the virtual objects collaboratively that objects are tracked in real-time by using the cameras. Moreover. These games are modeled to encourage natural communication and coordination between the users with the offered Communication-advancement mode that make user capable of information sharing and discuss the strategies of the game with the help of messages and voice communication. According to the practicability study with 12 ASD children and 12 normally developing peers, this system was nicely granted by both Normal children and ASD children, enhanced their coordination in the gameplay, and proved the ability for boosting their communication and coordination skills.

Dinstein et al. (2020) has selected a group of children recording who speak Hebrew and have undergone a session of Autism Diagnostic Observation Schedule (ADOS) assessment. From these recordings, he has concluded some characteristics based on the acoustic, prosodic and conversational characteristics. The total number of characteristics selected was 60 and out of these 72 recordings, 21 characteristics were completely related with the score of ADOS of the children. Zero-Crossing Rate (ZCR) was determined to calculate the correlations, and negative correlations were got with the number of vocal responses and speed to the clinician, and whole vocalizations number. Deriving the conclusive remarks from these outcomes the research was focused on the development of an artificial neural network with deep learning (Goyal et al., 2021) to estimate the score of ADOS and then it is subjected to the linear regression models along with the support vector machines. The comparative analysis on these three models concluded the efficiency of the convolution neural network to be best having the RMSE of 4.65 and mean correlation of 0.72 with the ADOS original data set during the training and prediction analysis.

4. DIAGNOSIS METHODS AND TOOLS

Behaviors observed in a child are often dependant on a count of non-autism distinct components, as well age and cognitive functioning so the appraisal of ASD can be complex.

The ASD diagnosis is further complex due to the interactions between ASD symptoms and development. Several features generally when informants defined are general to ASD are no strictly exclusive to the diagnosis and may occur in different disorders at the fixed age. According to Wang et al. (2018), a study by caretakers and parents, the popularity of the stereotyped language is less now in the children having ASD than in the children developing typically and different non-spectrum diagnoses children under the age of four and children without any difficult language (Kautish & Ahmed, 2016). These discoveries show that the kind of behavior to which a medical practitioner must attend for diagnosis is mostly dependent on the components of development such as language level and age, as well as the information source.

The current studies hold up a precise connection between motor system development. General movements (GMs) and crying could be recognized as early signs of neurodevelopment disorders since they are both connected to neurotransmission functionality in fixed areas of the brain (Reyana et al, 2020). These signs have been studied in many studies. Cry includes central nervous system activation and needs an equal exertion of various regions of the brain. Infants with neurological positions and preterm infants have distinct cry functions when differentiating to the healthy infants. Being completely contact-less and chap, cry inspection has currently excited interest as an early indication of probable disturbances central nervous system with ASDs. Many studies substantiate that newborn infants possessed by distinct brain lesions naturally lose fluency, elegance, and complexity. Although the inspection of carrying and movements perceptually has been finished in clinics with the specialty. For saving time and reducing the errors of clinicians, the absence of automated tools for the aim of ASD diagnosis and the high quality of its severity is needed (Girli et al., 2018).

For comparing the learning disability (LD) children and children with ASD with the help of body and the facial expression-based system was evolved by Girli et al. (2018). The author in Hayo et al. (2016) evolved a system for recognition of the emotion for autism spectrum children with many modalities in an expression like facial, body, and voice. Santhosh kumar et al. (2019) estimated simple emotions from children with ASD (autism spectrum disorder) with the help of movements of the body. For the prediction of emotions from the movements of the body, characteristics12dimensional movements of the body (distance, velocity, angle, and acceleration)from the head, L, and R hand are defined in this document. The recorded videos of autistic children (5-11 years, n=10) are the dataset for this observation. The fetched characteristics are specified to the Random Forest (RF) and the Support Vector Machine (SVM) classifier for children's emotions prediction. The method for detecting ASD using electroencephalography (EEG) and Eye-tracking (ET) is described by Black et al. (2017). The methodology will be useful for observing the neurological co-relation for distinct activities and also for representing the in contrast of normal behavior. The behavior typically developed (TD) children and ASD patients is explained by Chen et al. (2019) so various emotional expressions are inspected such as gazing of movements of eye and expressions of faces. developed a tool for inspection of autism rehabilitation, the author had evolved a game of computer for emotional state understanding. The model is practiced to understand emotions i.e., emergence, regulation, and recognition of emotions. For finding the algorithms for recognizing the patterns to screen ASD children, the game is capable for both normal and autistic children.

5. APPLICATION OF DEEP LEARNING FOR NEUROIMAGING

Artificial intelligence (AI) is an IT branch that includes machine learning, representation, and profound learning. In classification radiology, risks assessments, segmentation functions, diagnosis, prognoses and even prediction of therapeutic reaction have been proposed to an expanding range of clinical applications focused on machinery or deep learning and related to radiology.

The learning-based algorithms that also include the various forms of deep and machine learning architecture are the area of research for several scientists. They have focussed on the development of certain learning framework using these systems for processing the image of the brain that can come out to be fruitful in the classification of stroke, some of the psychiatric disorders, epilepsy, neuron degeneratively disorders, and demyelinating diseases

The portrayal of learning is being done by the neural networks that form an architectural arrangement of the most specific features that are then learned by the algorithm. The various forms of the neural architecture include the recurrent neural network abbreviated as RNN and the convolution neural network often referred to as CNN.

Several approaches have been recently proposed for deep learning image production and image improvement, from the elimination of image errors, standardization/harmonization of images, an image with improved and efficient quality followed by a reduction in radiation along with the contrast dose and imaging experiments lessening. The basic definition of machine learning can be explained as the algorithms comprising of the neural network frameworks working as supervised-based learning architecture or non-supervised learning system. It can also function as a semi-supervised based architecture of learning. There have been much researches on these learning frameworks but those associated with the efficient functioning of neuron imaging are still an obstacle. The first thing is that the fitting is completed. The possibility of overfitting is often posed by training a complex classifier with a limited data set. The researches are done to bring about the conclusion regarding the deep learning algorithms that, even though they can be easily fitted for the data knowledge, they are difficult to be generalized. The analysis of different techniques has been done via experimentation, including regularization, early stopping, and drops out, to minimize overfitting. Although overfitting may be measured by the algorithm output in a single data set, it could be difficult for the algorithm to perform well with identical pictures obtained in multiple centers on different scanners.

In general, larger data sets from numerous centers of different scanners and protocols are obtained in various ways that result in poor algorithm performance if subjected to slightly different images. It has been found that data increased cannot adequately solve problems with limited databases without standard requirements.

Solving this challenge, called "breakdown AI", is a significant research field if these methods are to be used extensively. Deep schooling is also a science of extreme data starvation. The algorithm makes use of enormous labeled example sets to attain the objective of achieving verified and effective performance levels for the clinical application. Large data sets are often difficult to deal with but for these algorithms, they are not extreme, since upstream applications such as image quality assurance learn mainly about a large number of image forecasts (where each person is assigned a single learning data point). However, it is necessary to create large, publicly labeled medical image databases, although privacy issues, costs, ground truth measurement, and label accuracy remain obstacles. One of the benefits of image acquisition applications is that data have already been marked in some way, whereby sampled or high-dose images are used for grading tasks. In addition to the ethical and legal problems, there is some trouble physiologically reading the effects of deep learning. Deep networks are "black boxes", in which data and a classification or picture performance forecast are produced (Jiang et al., 2019). There have been inferences of referring to the deep learning algorithms as "myths of modeling perception" due to their ability to act in higher dimensions when compared to the human brains (Moon et al., 2019). The understanding of the images generated can be improved by the prediction algorithms. The recent advancements in the field of machine learning algorithms have been able to pave the path for more precise analysis of radiology images. The process of image quality enhancement deploying these algorithms forms the initial stage of the development. In their early stages, deeper learning approaches still exist in medical imaging.

The interest in classification generalization with machine learning is developing in the field of neuron imaging. The method of the DL has been subjected to be utilized in the field of psychology in the form of a screening tool that aims at the classification of the risk of acquiring diseases in a high-risk group and as a predictive model of the reaction to therapy between the patient and the usual groups. Alzheimer's and moderate cognitive dysfunction were investigated on a variety of diagnostic models; however, the number of neural developmental disability trials is restricted. The study by the author made the classification based on heterogeneous illness group and found that in ASD n=98, whereas for ADHD n=930. Further, the classification was extended to derive post-traumatic stress disorder to be n=87 and Alzheimer's disease to be n=132 using classification using machine learning. In this analysis, 18 classifications of machine learning were introduced and their predictive powers combined to create a plan with a consensus classification. The functional relation pattern found had been firmly used for the determination of the differences associated with the method of classification along with the age and data acquisition areas. This also included the ability to discern statistically relevant differences between groups in diagnostic prediction. The method chosen for the testing primarily was magnetic resonance imaging (MRI) and then it was performed with the help of functional MRI (fMRI). The study was further extended to the near-infrared spectroscopy (fNIRS) that performed the tests based on the neuron-based imaging and DL methods for neuron developmental disorders. The majority of experiments are focused on the assessment of DL diagnostic specificity, and there are certain instances of examining the anatomical variations inside the brains of the patient group and compare them with the variations inside the normal group to bring about the early detection of the biomarkers.

Lanka et al. (2020) thoroughly evaluated and analyzed 40 ASD computer study algorithms released between 2007 and 2018. 0.83, was found to be the integrated sensitivity while the 0.84 were detected to be the specificity and the ratio of (AUC/pAUC) was found to be 0/90/0.83 which is defined as the area under curve divided by the partial area under the curve in the particular meta-analysis for 12 samples of structural residue. Based on this, the authors found the precision of the machine learning algorithm for ASD diagnosis with structural MRI that requires to be exact and proper.

Chen et al. (2019) used Dilated Dense U-Net as a new DL technique to find ASD neurobiological defects and verified the crucial progressive period of amygdala and hippocampus growth via longitudinal studies. 276 MRI longitudinal brain scans have been obtained in the NDAR (30 ASD, 31 medium autism spectra, and 215 NC groups). The presence of CA1-3 amygdala with bilateral expansion was found to be associated with the children who were 6 months old and detection of bilateral CA1-3 amygdala left were found to be at 24 months after the birth by the process of cross-analysis. CA1-3 left subicula expansion. Longitude analyses reveal that the ASD group has grown in size to about 6 months, with the size of the group at around 24 months, with bilateral amygdale and bilateral CA1-3. They proposed that the amygdala and CA1-3 over-growth from the age of 6 months may contribute to the possibility of determining the potential of ASD in children of age up to 6 months and detect them as early as possible. The research conducted by the Yoo et al. (2020) brought the conclusion that the process involving machine learning having multimode neurology with genetic evidence can be beneficial in categorizing the children that have been achieved by ADHD. The greatest precision and exactness achieved is 85.1 percent when referring to the model for cortical thickness and the volume model. There were instances of morphological differences present which was reported as the main predictors. The differences were also found in the ventral frontal cortex, comprising 18 percent of the ADHD scale. A continuous performance test (CPT) was performed to see a precision of 69.4% where 6.4% missed the errors in the test. There was complex zone homogeneity within the default network. Results of this research suggest that a strong classifier for ADHD diagnosis and the effects of structural anomalies associated with salience, auditory processing, and respiration suppression.

The confirmation regarding the diagnostics classifications drawn are making use of DL keeping the brain frequency at its peak has been achieved by the data of 198 ASD consisting of the children from school (Xiao et al., 2019). The overall accuracy of diagnosis is 96.26%, 98.03%, and 93.62% precision. These findings are more precise than prior tests, which only identified one to two frequency bands. This is up to 15 percent. This diagnostic precision is improved. In the reconstruction fMRI results for 5-10 years of age, ASD children are subject to CNN.

The model has been intended to be derived by making use of the ADHD-200 data collection for diagnosing a vector support machinery in a research carried out by Wang et al. (2018) (SVMs). LOOCV and 10-fold inter validation analyzed the efficiency of the diagnostic model (CV). LOOCV shows 78.75% precision, 76% accuracy, and 80.71% specificity of a model. The average accuracy of the 10-fold CV forecast was around 75,54±1,34 percent and the average sensitivity 70,5±2,34 percent. More researches that are being conducted in recent times have concluded the potential of the ADHD differential patterns as a biomarker when analyzed using the SVM method.

Neuron imaging experiments have indicated multiple biomarkers for neuron developmental disorders; however, the systematic study of these biomarkers has constraints that will yield clinically useful findings. The evidence for the clinical tests has been added on by the new method referred to as DL intended to assist in neuronal developmental disability recognition which has been developed from the sequential tests that are already existing. The key objective to bring about such methodology is to provide increased and efficient assistance to the lab technicians and improve the specificity of the diagnosis further.

6. PROPOSED METHODOLOGY

The existing ASD diagnosis tools are mostly based on behavior observation and symptoms which can be sometimes misdiagnosed. So, to develop a more qualitative diagnosis, there is a need for advanced tools and artificial intelligence interfaces to visualize and analyze the biological abnormalities for ASD disorders. In this work,

Figure 2. Clinical Decision Support System

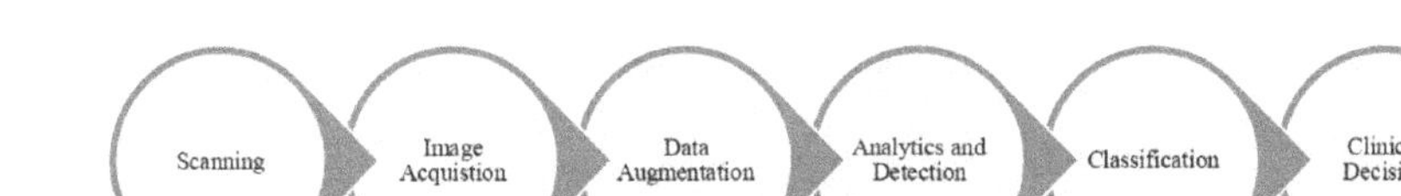

a framework is proposed using a deep learning-based image processing tool to classify ASD subjects from healthy subjects from neuroimages for clinical decision support (Fig. 2).

According to the study, one of the deep learning approaches, convolution neural network (CNN) is mostly used for image process as it has capabilities to classify complex problems and extract features from small image patches. The benefits of CNN have motivated the proposed architecture to incorporate CNN as the base model for ASD children's behavior analysis from neuroimages of the brain. The system architecture is illustrated in Fig. 3.

The proposed system will use functional and structural information from neuro-images and. These features are fused after dimension reduction of features by using any less complex dimension reduction techniques, such as principal component analysis (PCA). The reduced dimension features are fed in CNN blocks consisting of convolutional layers with small kernels, having a similar responsive field of one layer with bigger kernels. This proposed network is based on residual learning. As deep neural network training process sometimes results in a vanishing gradient problem. So, dimension reduction to remove irrelevant features will reduce this problem. The cost function (loss function) will be needed to be focused that increases the efficiency level while training very deep in the residual block.

Table 1 illustrates the theoretical comparison over existing works. The implementation of the proposed architecture will show improvement over existing techniques in terms of performance features and parameters.

7. CHALLENGES AND FUTURE RESEARCH DIRECTION

Many existing reviews or surveys are presented on autism spectrum disorder detection and remedial approaches to understanding the feelings of ASD suffering children using machine learning or deep learning approach. In this chapter different

Figure 3. The proposed framework for ASD diagnosis using neuro-images

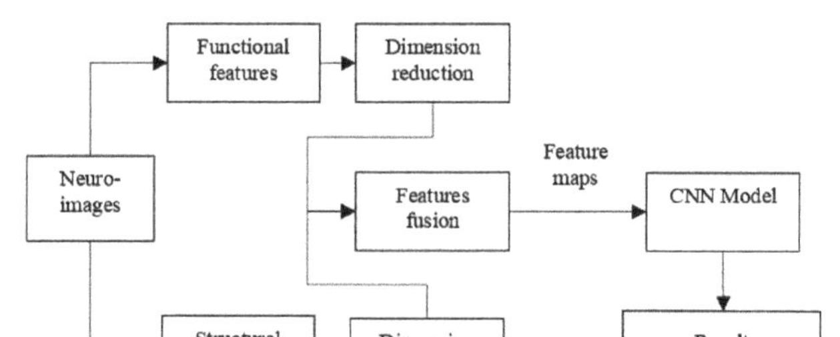

Algorithm 1. Proposed ASD framework

```
Input: MRI brain image data set (with label)
Output: ASD label (normal or Autistic)
Extract small structural and functional image patches from input MRI images.
Normalization across all patches.
Feature Dimension reduction
Feature fusion
Train using Residual CNN Model to determine the labels (classes).
For i= no of epochs
Determine the center voxel label of each patch from its ground Truth respectively.
Apply the Residual CNN Model
Minimize cost function
End for
For Testing Phase
Segment and classify each patient using the Residual CNN Model as follow:
extract patches
The model will predict classes (patches)
Reconstruct image from the Predicted patch
Compare reconstructed image and Original Ground Truth using performance evaluation metrics.
```

Table 1. Features comparison with existing techniques

Ref	Data	Technique	Features	Type	Parameters
Masood et al. (2020)	ASD screening	ML	functional	Binary	Accuracy
Akhondzadeh et al. (2020)	MRI	CNN	functional	Binary	Accuracy, Specificity, Sensitivity, F-score
Tao et al. (2019)	Eye movement	CNN-LSTM	Saliency maps	Binary	Accuracy
Jayawardana et al. (2019)	EEG	CNN	Temporal	Binary	Accuracy, Precision, recall, F1, R^2, MAE, RMSE
Sadouk et al. (2018)	EEG	CNN	Frequency and time domain	Binary	Accuracy, F1
Dvornek et al (2018)	FMRI	3D-CNN	spatial	Binary	F_score
Choi et al (2020)	MRI	3D-CNN	spatial	Binary	Accuracy
Wang et al. (2020)	fMRI	ML	singular value decomposition	Binary	Accuracy, Specificity, Sensitivity
Yang et al. (2019)	Image and Text	ML	Chi-squared	-	Precision, recall, F1
Proposed	MRI	CNN	Functional and structural	Multi classification	Accuracy, Specificity, Sensitivity, F-score, MAE, RMSE

Figure 4. Future Research Scopes

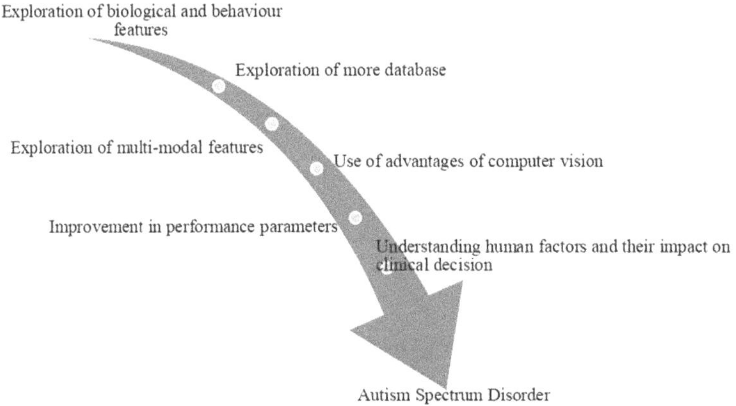

diagnosis approaches were explored, such as facial expressions, eye movements, EEG signals, and brain imaging. Out of all, brain imaging is a field in which not much research works are focused or achieved much accurate performance. Some major contributions of researchers in ASD diagnosis are stated in Table 2. There are no past works that have provided a profound discussion about neuroimaging as a base for ASD diagnosis. This chapter also provided a brief description of challenges and issues related to ASD diagnosis. To resolve these issues, this chapter also proposed architecture and also redirects the researchers towards future research scopes.

Due to current research, the following problems should be tackled by researchers in this area:

- Multimodal techniques focused on methods of multimodal fusion. Much of the studies currently concentrate on RGB image data or video streams. However, more and more studies have shown that a combination of multimodal knowledge will produce superior results.
- For more accurate performance comparison, future research works should be focused on a benchmark dataset such as (ABIDE) and test developed models on them. Specialists can take information from current state-of-the-art models of recognition of human behavior trained on neuro-image information, apply them to these datasets, and create models that can be applied to people with ASD.
- An application of computer vision has shown its efficiency in the unconstrained scenario.
- Most of the existing works are reported to require participants to be in clinical settings, that in their natural environments, usually do not collect data from children.

Table 2. Some existing diagnosis process

Diagnosis	Techniques	Result and Discussions	Ref
ASD Screening Data for Adult ASD Screening Data for Children ASD Screening Data for Adolescent	CNN	ASD and Non -ASD category evaluation. Handled missing values in the dataset. Achieved approx. 98% accuracy on binary classification.	Masood et al. (2020) Akhondzadeh et al. (2020) Tao et al. (2019)
ASD diagnosis using brain image dataset.	10-fold validation using CNN	Achieved accuracy of about 70.22%. The time complexity needed to be improved. Gender and age group was not considered for analysis.	Jayawardana et al. (2019)
Eye Movement dataset for ASD children	CNN-LSTM	When the images are natural scenes or no face is shown in the images, the model performs worse.	Sadouk et al. (2018)
ASD diagnosis using the EEG dataset.	CNN	Analyze the short-term and long-term relationships between ASD and brain activity using EEG.	Dvornek et al (2018)
Stereotypical motor movements (SMM) for ASD	CNN	The accuracy for binary classification was 95%.	Masood et al. (2020)
ASD diagnosis using brain fMRI	3-D CNN	The average F-scores obtained was 8.5%.	Akhondzadeh et al. (2020)
ASD diagnosis using brain MRI	CNN and RNN	Maximum accuracy of 90% at YUM dataset and 64% at ABIDE dataset.	Choi et al (2020)
ASD diagnosis using brain fMRI	Low-rank feature representation with KNN and SVM classifier.	Maximum accuracy of 75%.	Wang et al. (2020)
ASD diagnosis using brain fMRI	GA optimized SVM classifier	96% accuracy was achieved.	Yang et al. (2019)
ASD using the image and textual robotic interaction	Neighbor discovery in the image with identification of duplicate frames.	67% average precision and 46% recall.	Yang et al. (2020)
ASD diagnosis using brain sMRI	Biomarker Exploration with Recurrent Attention Model	Achieved 87% of accuracy.	Mostafa et al. (2019)
ASD diagnosis using brain fMRI	Eigenvalues	Achieved 77% of accuracy.	Rusli et al. (2020)

- To determine the efficiency of successful computer vision systems, research is needed to explore the feature correlation using computer vision techniques. To guarantee precision, reliability, interpretability, and true clinical usefulness requires careful and systematic empirical confirmation. This will help decide the unbiased result.
- There is a need to explore deep knowledge about the impact of human factors and ethical concerns integrated with computer vision that would help to build functional and useful tools and to decide whether these systems can be used in a clinical environment to increase current behavioral observations.

8. CONCLUSION

In this chapter, an overview of autism spectrum disorder is presented. As autism is categorized as a neuro-disorder in any person. Autism can be detected at any stage of life as a "behavioral diversion disease". Generally, autism problem starts from childhood and exists lifelong. With rising applications of computer vision and machine learning, this had led the advancements in the medical diagnosis field. This chapter is mainly focused on the exploration of machine learning or deep learning applications for ASD diagnosis. The chapter gives a brief description of the result analysis of existing techniques that concludes with the efficiency of the CNN model for ASD diagnosis. Thus, the proposed methodology uses the computer vision application and CNN model for diagnosis of ASD efficiently. In the proposed methodology, the fusion of structural features and functional features is used to more accurately diagnose ASD complexity. Certainly, due to fusion of two brain features will increase the training complexity but simultaneously this would reduce the training losses. So, in future work, there is room for reducing the learning complexity. The study also gives future research direction to use the advancement of digital image processing to develop a more feasible framework for accurate diagnosis of ASD subjects with the integration of deep learning.

REFERENCES

Black, M. H., Chen, N. T. M., Iyer, K. K., Lipp, O. V., Bölte, S., Falkmer, M., Tan, T., & Girdler, S. (2017). Mechanisms of facial emotion recognition in autism spectrum disorders: Insights from eye tracking and electroencephalography. *Neuroscience and Biobehavioral Reviews*, *80*, 488–515. doi:10.1016/j.neubiorev.2017.06.016 PMID:28698082

Del Coco, M., Leo, M., Carcagni, P., Fama, F., Spadaro, L., Ruta, L., Pioggia, G., & Distante, C. (2018). Study of Mechanisms of Social Interaction Stimulation in Autism Spectrum Disorder by Assisted Humanoid Robot. *IEEE Transactions on Cognitive and Developmental Systems*, *10*(4), 993–1004. doi:10.1109/TCDS.2017.2783684

Eni, M., Dinstein, I., Ilan, M., Menashe, I., Meiri, G., & Zigel, Y. (2020). Estimating Autism Severity in Young Children from Speech Signals Using a Deep Neural Network. *IEEE Access: Practical Innovations, Open Solutions*, *8*, 139489–139500. doi:10.1109/ACCESS.2020.3012532

Fridenson-Hayo, S., Berggren, S., Lassalle, A., Tal, S., Pigat, D., Bölte, S., Baron-Cohen, S., & Golan, O. (2016). Basic and complex emotion recognition in children with autism: Cross-cultural findings. *Molecular Autism*, *7*(1), 1–11. doi:10.118613229-016-0113-9 PMID:28018573

Girli, A., Doğmaz, S., & Fakültesi, E. (2018). Ability of Children with Learning Disabilities and Children with Autism Spectrum Disorder to Recognize Feelings from Facial Expressions and Body Language. *World J Educ*, *8*(2), 10. Advance online publication. doi:10.5430/wje.v8n2p10

Goyal, S. B., Bedi, P., Kumar, J., & Varadarajan, V. (2021). Deep learning application for sensing available spectrum for cognitive radio: An ECRNN approach. *Peer-to-Peer Networking and Applications*. Advance online publication. doi:10.100712083-021-01169-4

Irani, A., Moradi, H., & Vahid, L. K. (2018). Autism Screening Using a Video Game Based on Emotions. In *2018 2nd National and 1st International Digital Games Research Conference: Trends, Technologies, and Applications, DGRC 2018*. Institute of Electrical and Electronics Engineers Inc. 10.1109/DGRC.2018.8712053

Jayawardana, Y., Jaime, M., & Jayarathna, S. (2019). Analysis of temporal relationships between ASD and brain activity through EEG and machine learning. In *Proceedings - 2019 IEEE 20th International Conference on Information Reuse and Integration for Data Science, IRI 2019*. Institute of Electrical and Electronics Engineers Inc. 10.1109/IRI.2019.00035

Kaur, R., & Kautish, S. (2019). Multimodal sentiment analysis: A survey and comparison. *International Journal of Service Science, Management, Engineering, and Technology*, *10*(2), 38–58. doi:10.4018/IJSSMET.2019040103

Kautish, S., & Ahmed, R. K. A. (2016). A Comprehensive Review of Current and Future Applications of Data Mining in Medicine & Healthcare. *Algorithms*, *6*(8), 9.

Ke, F., Choi, S., Kang, Y. H., Cheon, K.-A., & Lee, S. W. (2020). Exploring the Structural and Strategic Bases of Autism Spectrum Disorders with Deep Learning. *IEEE Access: Practical Innovations, Open Solutions*, *8*, 153341–153352. doi:10.1109/ACCESS.2020.3016734

Ke, F., & Yang, R. (2020). Classification and Biomarker Exploration of Autism Spectrum Disorders Based on Recurrent Attention Model. *IEEE Access: Practical Innovations, Open Solutions*, *8*, 216298–216307. doi:10.1109/ACCESS.2020.3038479

Lanka, P., Rangaprakash, D., Dretsch, M. N., Katz, J. S., Denney, T. S. Jr, & Deshpande, G. (2020). Supervised machine learning for diagnostic classification from large-scale neuroimaging datasets. *Brain Imaging and Behavior*, *14*(6), 2378–2416. doi:10.100711682-019-00191-8 PMID:31691160

Li, G., Chen, M. H., Li, G., Wu, D., Lian, C., Sun, Q., Shen, D., & Wang, L. (2019). A Longitudinal MRI Study of Amygdala and Hippocampal Subfields for Infants with Risk of Autism. Lecture Notes in Computer Science (Including Subseries Lecture Notes in Artificial Intelligence and Lecture Notes in Bioinformatics), 11849, 164–171. doi:10.1007/978-3-030-35817-4_20

Li, X., Dvornek, N. C., & Papademetris, X. (2018) 2-Channel convolutional 3D deep neural network (2CC3D) for fMRI analysis: ASD classification and feature learning. In *Proceedings - International Symposium on Biomedical Imaging*. IEEE Computer Society.

Moon, S. J., Hwang, J., Kana, R., Torous, J., & Kim, J. W. (2019). Accuracy of machine learning algorithms for the diagnosis of autism spectrum disorder: Systematic review and meta-analysis of brain magnetic resonance imaging studies. Journal of Medical Internet Research, 21(12). doi:10.2196/14108

Mostafa, S., Tang, L., & Wu, F. X. (2019). Diagnosis of Autism Spectrum Disorder Based on Eigenvalues of Brain Networks. *IEEE Access: Practical Innovations, Open Solutions*, *7*, 128474–128486. doi:10.1109/ACCESS.2019.2940198

Raj, S., & Masood, S. (2020). Analysis and Detection of Autism Spectrum Disorder Using Machine Learning Techniques. In *Procedia Computer Science* (pp. 994–1004). Elsevier B.V. doi:10.1016/j.procs.2020.03.399

Rani, S., & Kautish, S. (2018). Application of data mining techniques for prediction of diabetes-A review. International Journal of Scientific Research in Computer Science. *Engineering and Information Technology*, *3*(3), 1996–2004.

Rani, S., & Kautish, S. (2018, June). Association clustering and time series based data mining in continuous data for diabetes prediction. In *2018 second international conference on intelligent computing and control systems (ICICCS)* (pp. 1209-1214). IEEE. 10.1109/ICCONS.2018.8662909

Reyana, A., & Kautish, S. (2021). *Corona virus-related Disease Pandemic: A Review on Machine Learning Approaches and Treatment Trials on Diagnosed Population for Future Clinical Decision Support*. Current Medical Imaging.

Reyana, A., Krishnaprasath, V. T., Kautish, S., Panigrahi, R., & Shaik, M. (2020). Decision-making on the existence of soft exudates in diabetic retinopathy. *International Journal of Computer Applications in Technology*, *64*(4), 375–381. doi:10.1504/IJCAT.2020.112684

Rusli, N., Sidek, S. N., Yusof, H. M., Ishak, N. I., Khalid, M., & Dzulkarnain, A. A. A. (2020). Implementation of Wavelet Analysis on Thermal Images for Affective States Recognition of Children with Autism Spectrum Disorder. *IEEE Access: Practical Innovations, Open Solutions*, *8*, 120818–120834. doi:10.1109/ACCESS.2020.3006004

Sadouk, L., Gadi, T., & Essoufi, E. H. (2018). A Novel Deep Learning Approach for Recognizing Stereotypical Motor Movements within and across Subjects on the Autism Spectrum Disorder. *Computational Intelligence and Neuroscience*, *2018*, 1–16. Advance online publication. doi:10.1155/2018/7186762 PMID:30111994

Sampathkumar, A., Rastogi, R., Arukonda, S., Shankar, A., Kautish, S., & Sivaram, M. (2020). An efficient hybrid methodology for detection of cancer-causing gene using CSC for micro array data. *Journal of Ambient Intelligence and Humanized Computing*, *11*(11), 4743–4751. doi:10.100712652-020-01731-7

Santhoshkumar, & Kalaiselvi Geetha. (2019). Emotion Recognition System for Autism Children using Non-verbal Communication. *International Journal of Innovative Technology and Exploring Engineering*, *8*(8), 159-165.

Sherkatghanad, Z., Akhondzadeh, M., Salari, S., Zomorodi-Moghadam, M., Abdar, M., Acharya, U. R., Khosrowabadi, R., & Salari, V. (2020). Automated Detection of Autism Spectrum Disorder Using a Convolutional Neural Network. *Frontiers in Neuroscience*, *13*, 1325. doi:10.3389/fnins.2019.01325 PMID:32009868

Su, Q., Chen, F., & Li, H. (2019). Multimodal emotion perception in children with autism spectrum disorder by eye tracking study. In *2018 IEEE EMBS Conference on Biomedical Engineering and Sciences, IECBES 2018 - Proceedings*. Institute of Electrical and Electronics Engineers Inc.

Tao, Y., & Shyu, M. L. (2019). SP-ASDNet: CNN-LSTM based ASD classification model using observer scanpaths. In *Proceedings - 2019 IEEE International Conference on Multimedia and Expo Workshops, ICMEW 2019*. Institute of Electrical and Electronics Engineers Inc.

Wang, M., Zhang, D., Huang, J., Yap, P.-T., Shen, D., & Liu, M. (2020). Identifying Autism Spectrum Disorder with Multi-Site fMRI via Low-Rank Domain Adaptation. *IEEE Transactions on Medical Imaging*, *39*(3), 644–655. doi:10.1109/TMI.2019.2933160 PMID:31395542

Wang, X. H., Jiao, Y., & Li, L. (2018). Identifying individuals with attention deficit hyperactivity disorder based on temporal variability of dynamic functional connectivity. *Scientific Reports*, *8*(1), 1–12. doi:10.103841598-018-30308-w PMID:30087369

Xiao, Z., Wu, J., Wang, C., Jia, N., & Yang, X. (2019). Computer-aided diagnosis of school-aged children with ASD using full frequency bands and enhanced SAE: A multi-institution study. *Experimental and Therapeutic Medicine*, *17*(5), 4055. doi:10.3892/etm.2019.7448 PMID:31007742

Yang, X., Shyu, M. L., Yu, H. Q., Sun, S.-M., Yin, N.-S., & Chen, W. (2019). Integrating image and textual information in human–robot interactions for children with autism spectrum disorder. *IEEE Transactions on Multimedia*, *21*(3), 746–759. doi:10.1109/TMM.2018.2865828

Yoo, J. H., Kim, J. I., Kim, B. N., & Jeong, B. (2020). Exploring characteristic features of attention-deficit/hyperactivity disorder: Findings from multi-modal MRI and candidate genetic data. *Brain Imaging and Behavior*, *14*(6), 2132–2147. doi:10.100711682-019-00164-x PMID:31321662

Zhao, H., Swanson, A. R., Weitlauf, A. S., Warren, Z. E., & Sarkar, N. (2018). Hand-in-Hand: A Communication-Enhancement Collaborative Virtual Reality System for Promoting Social Interaction in Children with Autism Spectrum Disorders. *IEEE Transactions on Human-Machine Systems*, *48*(2), 136–148. doi:10.1109/THMS.2018.2791562 PMID:30345182

Zheng, Z., Young, E. M., Swanson, A. R., Weitlauf, A. S., Warren, Z. E., & Sarkar, N. (2016). Robot-Mediated Imitation Skill Training for Children with Autism. *IEEE Transactions on Neural Systems and Rehabilitation Engineering*, *24*(6), 682–691. doi:10.1109/TNSRE.2015.2475724 PMID:26353376

Zhu, G., Jiang, B., Tong, L., Xie, Y., Zaharchuk, G., & Wintermark, M. (2019). Applications of deep learning to neuro-imaging techniques. *Frontiers in Neurology*, *10*(Aug), 869. doi:10.3389/fneur.2019.00869 PMID:31474928

Chapter 2
A Novel Neuro-Fuzzy System-Based Autism Spectrum Disorder

Rubal Jeet
Chandigarh Engineering College, India

Mohammad Shabaz
Chitkara University, India

Garima Verma
DIT University, India

Vinay Kumar Nassa
https://orcid.org/0000-0002-9606-7570
South Point Group of Institutions, Sonepat, India

ABSTRACT

The major purpose of these research works has been for the rapid, reliable diagnosis of autism disorder by a new neuro-fuzzy autism identification technique. The highly affected region for each person is highlighted by this procedure. This research, which involves autism and regular group, included two classes of adolescents. This neuro-fuzzy method was developed by the experts using fuzzy-logical principles. The two classes were checked on the system. The developed method has been confirmed to distinguish easily between autistic participants and normal participants with increased precision. The engineered device has also been found to be 97.3% precise and 98.9% specific. The engineered instrument can be used by physicians to diagnose autism in conjunction with the seriousness of autism and to precisely and immediately illuminate the highly affected region.

DOI: 10.4018/978-1-7998-7460-7.ch002

INTRODUCTION

Autism is an early developmental neurodevelopment disorder that is fully characterized by three disorders, including social contact, voice and repetitive or typically stereo behaviour. In 1943 the word "autism" was coined by Dr. Kanner, University of John Hopkins. Autism is not an uncommon pathology since it is the third most common psychiatric disease in the world. Recent population data show that autism rises rapidly per 1 out of 68 children globally, and diagnostic and intervention are very high every year (Weksberg et. al., 2013).

Data on an outbreak of ball parks in India is not available and the majority of children in India who have not been diagnosed with autism are not cared for. This problem occurs in many developing countries, but is particularly true in India in which qualified physicians do not know how to detect or diagnose the illness, as the conventional diagnosis technique is not available. To date, there has been no autism cure. Many therapies, however, allow children with autism to improve their quality of life. Two important aspects are early intervention and extremely formal programmed that offer the greatest chance for progress for children with autism. Early diagnosis thus appearing as the cause of some positive results, including beginning early intervention, decreasing family burdens, reducing social costs, and prior association of the major autism impairments in physical, behavioral and psychological conditions.

There are conventional screening and testing instruments, such as Autism in Checkers (CHAT), Autism Diagnostic Interview Revised (ACR) and Autism Autism Rating Scale (ADI-R), Second edition (PDDST-II), Modified Autism in Toddler (M-CHAT). Additional types of scanning instruments are also used (DSM-V).

The ASD is a general neuro-sophisticated condition. There are many illnesses in combination, including intellectual disabilities, convulsions and anxieties (Hochberg et. al.,1995). In the 2013 survey 1 of 6-17-year-olds found ASD (Manzardo et. al., 2015). SSDs have moderate to extremely difficult contacts and coordination and have restricted, repetitive behaviour and concerns (Weksberg et. al., 2013). The precision of ASD patients under conventional controls is a crucial step (TC). Currently, multi brain treatment technology, such as ASD and schizophrenia, have been used widely for the treatment of multiple brain disorders (Vahia, 2013), (Geschwind etc., 2011).

One of the primary causes of hospitalization is the self-injurious behaviour of children with autism (ASD) (Kalb et al., 2016). The SIB can be rhythmic and repeated and involves behaviour like knockouts (Minshawi et al., 2014). SIB can cause physical damage, including abrasion, laceration and bruising (Rooker et al. 2018), particularly when SIB normally goes beyond its initial age. Early interventions will, however, help minimize severe problems and long-term continuity of SIB (Kurtz et al., 2003).

The magnet resonance imaging technology (MRI), which provides high-resolution 3D brain structure representations and precise structural data, is a powerful and safe technique. Morphological studies on the basis of MRI pictures achieved promising results for the related diseases. The results have shown, in order to conduct the ASD classification and achieve successful classification effectiveness (Wange 2017), the variable brain and cerebral variability are correlated with geographic cortical thicknesses based on ASD with six pre-selected volume-related performing characteristics. For example. For example. The morphological features of MRI data to characterize schizophrenia were collected (Brown et al.2013), including a medium cortical diameter, geographical cortical mass, etc. (Sahin et al.2018), and shown that the frontal lobe grey matter is lower in the normal controls in schizophrenic patients (Sahin et al. 2013) Schizophrenia (Craig et. al., 2008).

Autism Spectrum Disorder (ASD) is a polygenetically evolving mental and behavioral mutilation brain disorder (Liu et. al., 2014). It is a lifetime neurodevelopmental disorder that demonstrates expression failures, interactions, and limited behaviour. Though ASD is mostly distinguished by social physiognomy and performed, autistic individuals may have impaired motor skills such as less physical synchro physics, unstable body coordination and erratic behaviour and position (Wagner et. al., 2015). Individuals with ASD experience traditional recurring behaviors, limited wishes, lack of instincts, voice impairments, diminished intellect and cognitive capabilities with respect to normal developing adolescents (TD). ASD was notoriously diagnosed with movie physiognomies (Abowd et. al., 2012).

Several approaches have been used for artificial intelligence to diagnose autism. Synchronization of fuzzy, the likelihood of the discrete wavelet transformation between the brain regions was examined. These characteristics were finally used to create a detailed autism diagnosis dependent on detected properties of autism and natural EEG functional connectivity. The exactness of this approach was some 95.4%, but the doctors did not use it due to complicated treatment and expensive equipment specifications. The model was a fuzzy model for carrying out the evaluation using a TSK inference engine. A first-order approach was used with a series of real-time data and the test findings were correlated with the conventional autism form of assessment. The findings show that the approach predicted succeeded well in determining the autism cut-off of 78,9 percent between the autistic groups. A developmental chart and a method of predicting children autism have been implemented and 82.5 percent have been accurately found. In an evaluation of the autism, the author suggested a classification paradigm for Parallel Neural Fuzzy (PNF). A nerve network has been trained to mimic skills when a theoretical awareness is implanted into the fugitive structure. The planned framework was approximately 72 per cent accurate but was not easy to use. This paper draws the characteristics of EEG signals and uses adaptive artificial intelligence systems to characterizes it.

Therefore, it was found that most of the procedures were not reliable and therefore were not easy to use, i.e., they were technically very technical and were impossible for doctors to use. Thus, the implementation of certain tools was required, which would be easy to use, reliable, time intensive, and also highlight significant affected areas, in order to be able to schedule treatments as required. The goal of this current research is to create and validate an exact, user-friendly graphical interface based on a fleeting hierarchical model in an autism evaluation, especially with a single grading based on each region of disability. Relevant action must also be taken into account, not general interventions. The diseases in autism are categorized as "parasites," five conditions are referred to as pervasive disorders (PDD). The most common three PDDs are autism, Asperger syndrome and coarsenic disease (PDD-NOS) Any of the most common conditions of growth include a childhood disintegration and Rett syndrome. Because any genetic condition has become extremely rare, and disease is now deemed not really to be part of the autism spectrum.

RELATED WORK

(Abowd et. al., 2012) neuro-fuzzying model has been developed to predict children's autism and the precision of the basic behave impairments has been found to be about 90%. The author used a fuzzy simulation technique Takagi–Sugeno Kang (TSK) focused on subtractive clustered features with electroencephalography (EEG). The planned machine had a precision of around 80. In this study, author has been using the Fuzzy-Synchronization Likelihood (FSL) technique for the interpretation of functional communication in children with autism.

(Wall et. al., 2015) proposed an immersive video game to improve intelligibility in the voice of autistic children. Autism is clearly not being dealt with. To help autistic children improve their skills through games and educational facilities. The Santos investigates in 2013 the first detection of autism, namely that patient signals during adolescent years are taken from the preverbal vocalization by using classification strategies controlled SVM (support vector machine). Chaminade is a shot started in 2012 that includes the use of MRI for young adults with a humanoid robot.

(Langley et. al., 2013) gesticulation is used to evaluate atypical fluctuations with and without ASD in the facial expressions of infants. Six face reactions have been securitized using knowledge theory, statistical simulation and time series modelling. Researchers have recently used data mining to improve and implement ASD diagnostic methods. The classification possibility in the various fields has proved to be an efficient computer learning. Therefore, some literatures have used machine learning tools to categories neural and behaviour indicators that discriminate against people with or without ASD. The strength of the eye to classify children's clusters with high or low ASD risk. Computer methods such as the 0.72 accurate, 0.69 vector accuracy system support sample and 0.89 linear discriminatory analysis accuracy have been implemented. In 2016 Bone gathered data from Autism Diagnostic Interview-Revised and Social Reaction Scales and used SVM's apprenticeship rating to have positive results for a significant individual with or without ADS.

(Wong et. al., 2001) the implementation of thc autism development of a predictive model was done by using a dataset of 32 potential risk elements (ANN). The artificial neural network's predictor exactness is 88%. Their studies encouraged and promoted the use of ANN for diagnosing ASD as an excellent procedure. 96.7 percent for SVM was the highest classification accuracy to date.

(Radhakrishna et al., 2019) examines issues of classification of non-standardized text by computer training techniques. ASD is suggested to be a terribly heterogeneous disorder, with subgroups with entirely different genetic expression signatures because of grouping. In order to increase grouping, it can be useful to stratify ASD subgroups and to increase input provided by clinical interventions.

(Graham et. al., 2019) Laplace uses a quick Bayesian logistics regression approach to avoid sparse text data predictive models before fitting it. They use this technique to scatter paper ratings and demonstrate that they produce lightweight models that are just as reliable as those that are compact in combination with feature selection, generated by vector classification aids or regression of the framework logistics.

(Abowd et. al., 2012) the estimation procedures were suggested in a group of kids with autism after three years of clinical assessment, operation and psychological treatment. In particular, the studies of infant prognosis of autism have been carried out with psychiatric, behavioral, social, and demographic approaches. You sought to forecast and identify behavioral and personal symptoms for short-term autism outcomes. Initially, data are obtained from lists of autism controls, the aberrant behaviour control list, using Naive Bayes algorithms, the general linear model, the logistic regression and the decision tree (Reyana et al, 2020). The findings were then proportionally positive or negative to the frequency of the clinical variables. The decision tree they used to show the data is used. This approach helps psychiatrists to find patients, even though there are interim findings, in sub-groups of autism and other complex neurodevelopment disabilities. Decision trees are trees for grouping purposes. An immediate element and each branch's product are represented by a tree node. The roads describe classification legislation. It is a reality that the decision-making authorities will imagine the evidence.

(Sahin, 2018) proof device for body-accelerometer sensors for data acquisition, simulation and auto-stimulation compliance. Initially, pathologic behavioral automated indexing was feasible, based on the findings of their synthetic evidence (Kaur & Kautish, 2019). They use the Marcov Modeled (HMM) to track seven tunings from the recorded accelerometer, including hand swing and body rocking.

Synthetic pathologic activity evidence on stable adult neurotypes is obtained. Their solution offers remote and continuous accuracy speeds.

(Wang, 2017) proposed monitoring scheme for dictionary generation based on characteristics and the clustering of higher order statistics (HOS). In addition, the computer was trained by semi-monitored techniques to create templates for current events using a subset of training information to learn about new events. The other portion of the data was used for the detection of new occurrences both in HOS and LPC. The algorithm proposed produced comparable results with the previously reported findings based on the supervised approach of initial dictionary education. The method is very difficult despite promising precise speeds, which limit the use of SMM detection.

Fuzzy Logic

In 1965, the concept of "fuzzy logic" was introduced with the proposal of a 1965 principle of Lotfi A. Zadeh fuzzy. The logic of Fuzzy has been applied in numerous areas from the control theory of artificial intelligence. Fuzzy logic may be a kind of very precious logic. The idea is approximate, not accurate, rather than fixed. Logical fluctuations with a reality in between 0 and 1 degrees. To contend with this, the angry rationale is extended, where Truth Wert is in the spectrum between entirely true and completely false. Specific functionalities control these degrees before language variables are used. Figure 1 shows the layout of Fuzzy logic.

Neuro-Fuzzy System

Fuzzy reasoning is like the mechanism of feeling and inference of the human being (Reyana, & Kautish (2021), (Rani, & Kautish (2018). In the form of structural if

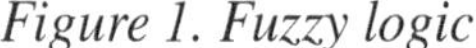

Figure 1. Fuzzy logic

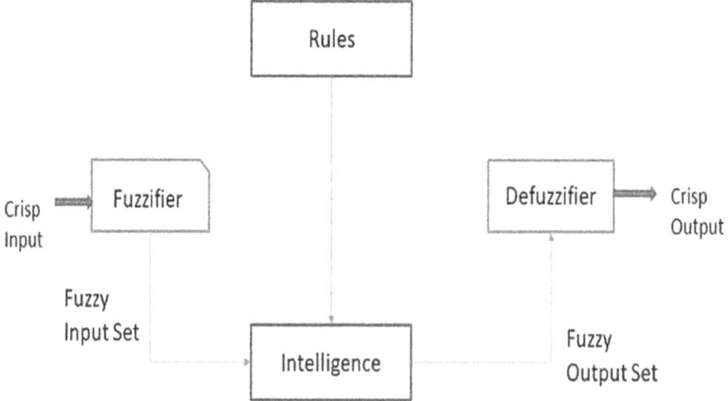

afterwards rules, a fuzzed inference scheme (FIS) effectively models the skills of specialist for a particular problem. In a wide range of areas such as decision making, pattern analysis, data classification etc., FIS applications are immense. The fuzzy theory offers a methodological means of linguistically signifying knowledge by making computational calculations using these linguistic labels for an inference process. These structures are known as Fuzzy Rule-Based (FRB). FRB is generally a protracted task requiring several stages, for example the learning of information, the specification of the controller, rules, and so on.

The number of laws is multiplied exponentially, since in conventional fuzzy schemes the number of the input part improves. If for and variable x variables and y membership functions are defined, y rules are needed to build a whole FRB structure. As x increases, the rule base easily strains the memory and runs the FRB process with difficulty. In fact, the obscurity of a problem exponentially increases with the input variables known as the dimensionality curse. Consequently, in dealing with the "dimensionality curse" and rules-explosion issue, the theory of Neuro Fuzzy Systems (NFSs) has been taken into account The HFSs are a set of low-dimensional, hierarchically formed fluid structures. The HFSs benefit from the fact that only the number of ingoing variables is matched by all laws.

Standard diagnostic models usually mark the child as "ordinary" or "abnormal" without affecting the accuracy or duration or diagnosis of aggregate CS. A diagnostic tool (Sampathkumar et al, 2020) that is accurate and fast and simple to use, that classifies autistic conditions as "normal," "small," "moderate" and "severe" was the main aim of this research study. The study also highlighted the child's highly affected environment. If the input variable numbers are higher, the major advantage of HFS is to reduce the number of rules substantially. Each module has its own configuration and the output of one module, based on the hierarchical architecture, is related to the next module's input.

Design of a Fuzzy-Based Module

This section outlines the implementation of each fuzzy module for the work currently undertaken. A collection of rules combined to describe the knowledge as if they were semantics. The whole process is divided into five separate sections, each with its own purpose. The various types of modules were designed: input, neuro-fuzzy, inference, defuzzification and decision. The selected 22 features with 22 attributes have been represented. These are attributes used as precursors to rules and each function (symptom) f. The extent of the child's role is every term {mild, moderate, rare}. If a child is, for example, unable to "only pay attention," a clinician will measure his level of presence as 4 and the device will designate "High (Always)" as the linguistic variable. "High (Always)" In decimals such as 1.4, 5.4, and 2.7

etc. the clinician also determined the severity of the boy. The input module sets a symptom vector to 22 attribute values and forward them to a fluid module.

An 'Si' attribute fluctuated with a 'xi' using a trapezoidal fuzzifier Each Xi variable in an output feature is mapped with the μ (Xi) membership feature into a value of 0 to 1. The attributes are hierarchically flushed and then add to an inference module deduction method to make an assessed reasoning. All the rules are in Mamdani format in this module and the resulting function returns a 'Yi' output. The Performance Module consists of four different classes of output: normal, gentle, modest and severe for various disorder stages. The winner is the highest score for the success class in the judgement module, and then the child is graded.

The lower engine uses the fluctuating equations to measure the regulation rules in the rule basis depending on the weight of the rule. Fuzzy inference is the process by which fuzzy logic is used to trace the input and output. The relation matrix was used to make all laws. The main logic behind this proposed approach is to determine the actual contribution to the severity of the disorder of each symptom and to mold it. The centroid process is used to defuse the output. The center of gravity or field system can be often referred to as this.

Dataset

For this article, Dataset was collected from the free UCI Research Repository (Murthy, 2001). Autistic data on child, 292 case and 21 characteristics, including age, race and patient nationality, were used in the survey. A Yaundice birth problem occurred, a family member had a large production disability, who did the experiment? The house where the customer is located, historically used screening systems for the consumer, scan procedures, multi-variate score, sample-based reaction.

Implementation

Two research groups, autism as the experimental population and regular control groups, were part of the research. Prior to this job, both parents and guardians received informed written consent. Participants from various special schools in Jalandhar were recruited. Prior to beginning the job, a meeting was held with each parent/keeper and child to offer an understanding of the actions of the study.

This trial involved 40 DT subjects, i.e. 28 males and 12 females; mean age 44 months and 40 participants from the autism community, i.e. 29 male and 11 female; average age 43.8 months. The difference in age between TD and autism ($p<0.002$) participants was not important. Both children with ASD were diagnosed with autism in accordance with DSM-IV guidelines. In addition, Autism Diagnostic Interview-

Figure 2. Neuro-Fuzzy system for ASD detection

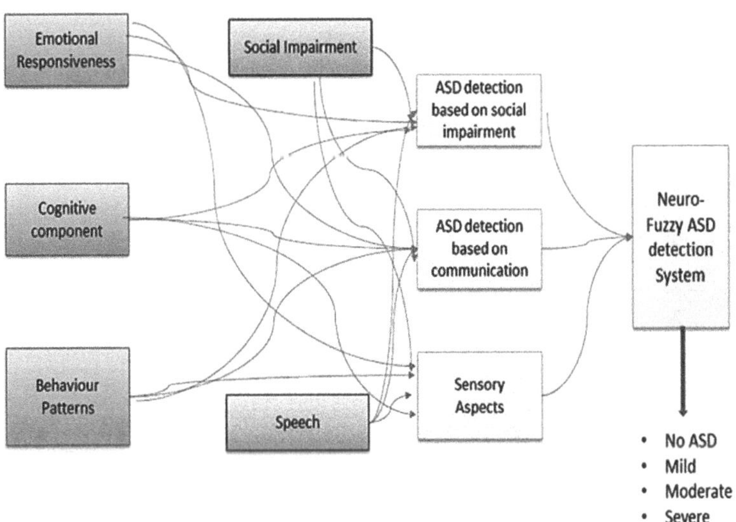

Revised (ADI-R) guidelines for ASD were complied with by each child with autism. Normal sexes and TD members of mental age were voluntary workers with no history of neurological disabilities. All participants were dextral and normally visualized or corrected. At the trial no child got any psychoactive drug. Figure 2 shows the Neuro-Fuzzy system for ASD detection.

RESULTS AND DISCUSSION

The mean values of the autism population were found to be considerably higher than the average. Statistically important mean variations have occurred ($p<0.001$). The mathematical null hypothesis is thus dismissed. CARS noticed similar patterns, but with less precision, longer time and a manual approach. On any of the six fields, the mean values were statistically different between the two sample groups.

This differentiates distinctly between autism and non-autistic participants and thus demonstrates their validity. Discriminant analysis was undertaken to assess the proper classification of the percentage of autism and normal children. The discrimination study assessed how reliably autism cases in the usual control category could be discriminated against.

The studies have shown that 98.7% of autistic and normal children have been properly classified. Similarly, a discriminant study has assessed how reliably CARS can discriminate cases of autism in the usual test category and has shown that 95.5%

Table 1. Linguistic states for automatic mode

Sr. No.	Variables	Values
1	Low	0-2.0
2	Medium	2.1-4.0
3	High	4.1-5.0

Table 2. Discriminant analysis using Neuro-Fuzzy system

Group	Predicted Group		
	Autism	Normal	Total
Autism	32	5	37
Normal	0	42	42
Autism	95	3	98
Normal	0	12	12

Table 3. Results of Neuro-Fuzzy system for ASD

Metrics	Result
Precision	97.3
Specificity	98.9

of autistic and normal children have been classified properly 96% was responsive and 97.8% were specific. For the same study, CARS were found to be less precise than in sample 03 autism-detected participants.

In order to assess its efficacy in discrimination of autistic and non-autistic people relative to CARS, sensitivity and precision have been measured. The system has 97.3% precision and 98.9% specificity. Sensitivity refers to the scale's ability to accurately recognize real autism cases as cases. Specificity applies to the scale's capacity to detect non-autists as non-cases properly. On CARS, the autism diagnosis score is reduced to 32. At 15.2 to 42.8, various sensitivity and specificity ranges were calculated with separated ratings. Distribution of the Linguistic states is given in Figure 3. Whereas, predicted values and results of precision and specificity are shown in Figure 4 and Figure 5 respectively. Details of Linguistic states for automatic mode is given in Table 1. The details for discriminant analysis using Neuro-Fuzzy system are provided in Table 2. And, Table 3 shows the results of Neuro-Fuzzy system for ASD.

Figure 3. Linguistic states

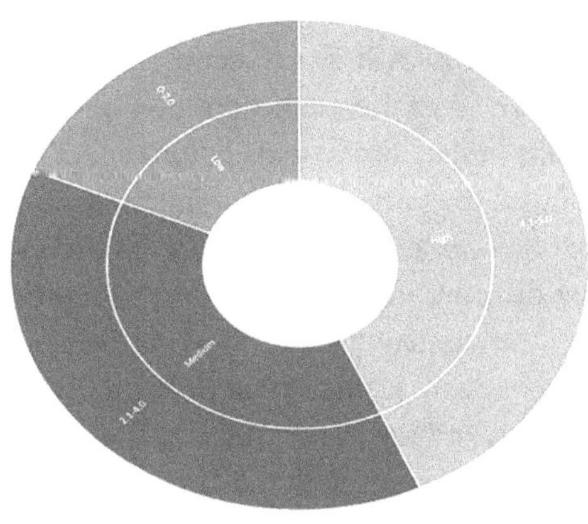

Figure 4. Predicted values

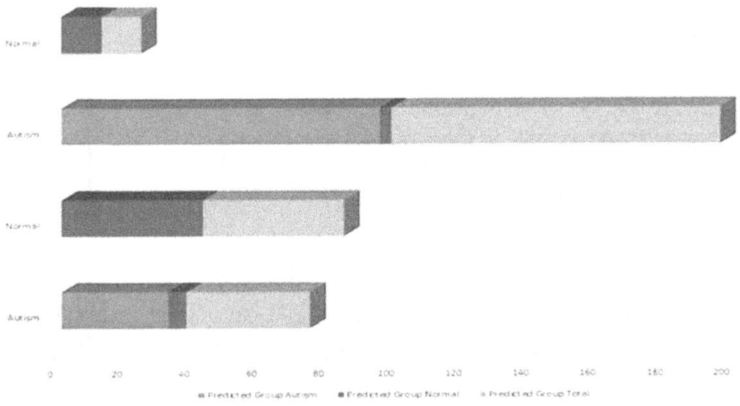

Figure 5. Results of precision and specificity

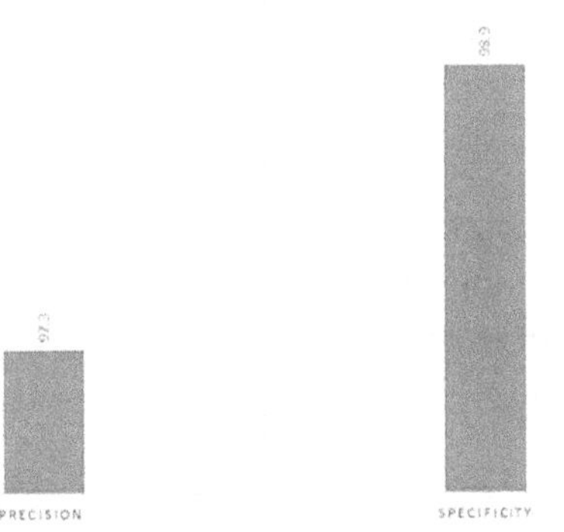

CONCLUSION

Autism continuum disturbances (ASDs) are identified by lack of social functioning and expression, in the face of limited concentration and repetitive behavior. The behavioral manifestations in the above fields before age 30 can be diagnosed with autism. Autism And autism are very difficult to identify because parents normally notice something about their infancy. Whilst many children with brain dysfunction and visual and hearing disorder in this group are overrepresented, many children suffer from autism have developmental impairment and behavioral delay. Persons that suffer from Asperger-like autism have normal or higher than average intelligence. The paper discusses autism and the many manifestations of autism and compares the efficiency of popular informatics with the fleeting thinking of the neuro-fuzzy method. The results of this analysis suggest that the psychometric properties of the neuro-fuzzy mechanism are strong. The method for evaluating autism is accurate and true.

REFERENCES

Bahado-Singh, R. O., Vishweswaraiah, S., Aydas, B., Mishra, N. K., Guda, C., & Radhakrishna, U. (2019). Deep learning / artificial intelligence and blood-based DNA epigenomic prediction of cerebralpalsy. *International Journal of Molecular Sciences*, 20. PMID:31035542

Bahado-Singh, R.O., Yilmaz, A., Bisgin, H., Turkoglu, O., Kumar, P., Sherman, E., Mrazik, A., Odibo, A., & Graham, S.F. (2019). Artificial intelligence and the analysis of multiplatform metabolomics data for the detection of intrauterine growth restriction. *PLoSOne, 14*.

Bengio, Y. (2009). Learning deep architectures for AI. Found. Trends®. *Machine Learning*, *2*(1), 1–127. doi:10.1561/2200000006

Benjamini, Y., & Hochberg, Y. (1995). Controlling the false discovery rate: A practical and powerful approach to multiple testing. *Journal of the Royal Statistical Society. Series B. Methodological*, *57*(1), 289–300. doi:10.1111/j.2517-6161.1995.tb02031.x

Butler, M. G., Rafi, S. K., Hossain, W., Stephan, D. A., & Manzardo, A. M. (2015). Whole exome sequencing in females with autism implicates novel and candidate genes. *International Journal of Molecular Sciences*, *16*(1), 1312–1335. doi:10.3390/ijms16011312 PMID:25574603

Chen, Y. A., Lemire, M., Choufani, S., Butcher, D. T., Grafodatskaya, D., Zanke, B. W., Gallinger, S., Hudson, T. J., & Weksberg, R. (2013). Discovery of cross-reactive probes and polymorphic CpGs in the Illumina Infinium Human Methylation 450 microarray. *Epigenetics*, *8*(2), 203–209. doi:10.4161/epi.23470 PMID:23314698

John, G. H., & Langley, P. (2013). *Estimating continuous distributions in Bayesian classifiers*. arXiv preprint arXiv:1302.4964.

Kaur, R., & Kautish, S. (2019). Multimodal sentiment analysis: A survey and comparison. *International Journal of Service Science, Management, Engineering, and Technology*, *10*(2), 38–58. doi:10.4018/IJSSMET.2019040103

Kosmicki, J. A., Sochat, V., Duda, M., & Wall, D. P. (2015). Searching for a minimal set of behaviors for autism detection through feature selection-based machine learning. *Translational Psychiatry*, *5*(2), e514–e514. doi:10.1038/tp.2015.7 PMID:25710120

Liu, B., Ma, Y., & Wong, C. K. (2001). Classification using association rules: weaknesses and enhancements. In *Data mining for scientific and engineering applications* (pp. 591–605). Springer. doi:10.1007/978-1-4615-1733-7_30

Plötz, T., Hammerla, N. Y., Rozga, A., Reavis, A., Call, N., & Abowd, G. D. (2012). Automatic assessment of problem behavior in individuals with developmental disabilities. *Proceedings of the 2012 ACM conference on ubiquitous computing*. 10.1145/2370216.2370276

Plötz, T., Hammerla, N. Y., Rozga, A., Reavis, A., Call, N., & Abowd, G. D. (2012). Automatic assessment of problem behavior in individuals with developmental disabilities. *Proceedings of the 2012 ACM conference on ubiquitous computing*. 10.1145/2370216.2370276

Poliker, R. (2006). Pattern recognition. In *Wiley Encyclopedia of biomedical engineering*. Wiley. doi:10.1002/9780471740360.ebs0904

Poliker, R. (2006). Pattern recognition. In *Wiley Encyclopedia of biomedical engineering*. Wiley. doi:10.1002/9780471740360.ebs0904

Preece, S. J., Goulermas, J. Y., Kenney, L. P., Howard, D., Meijer, K., & Crompton, R. (2009). Activity identification using body-mounted sensors - A review of classification techniques. *Physiological Measurement*, *30*(4), R1–R33. doi:10.1088/0967-3334/30/4/R01 PMID:19342767

Rani, S., & Kautish, S. (2018). Application of data mining techniques for prediction of diabetes-A review. International Journal of Scientific Research in Computer Science. *Engineering and Information Technology*, *3*(3), 1996–2004.

Rani, S., & Kautish, S. (2018, June). Association clustering and time series based data mining in continuous data for diabetes prediction. In *2018 second international conference on intelligent computing and control systems (ICICCS)* (pp. 1209-1214). IEEE. 10.1109/ICCONS.2018.8662909

Reyana, A., & Kautish, S. (2021). *Corona virus-related Disease Pandemic: A Review on Machine Learning Approaches and Treatment Trials on Diagnosed Population for Future Clinical Decision Support.* Current Medical Imaging.

Reyana, A., Krishnaprasath, V. T., Kautish, S., Panigrahi, R., & Shaik, M. (2020). Decision-making on the existence of soft exudates in diabetic retinopathy. *International Journal of Computer Applications in Technology*, *64*(4), 375–381. doi:10.1504/IJCAT.2020.112684

Saini, G. K., Chouhan, H., Kori, S., Gupta, A., Shabaz, M., Jagota, V., & Singh, B. K. (2021). Recognition of Human Sentiment from Image using Machine Learning. *Annals of the Romanian Society for Cell Biology*, *25*(5), 1802–1808.

Sampathkumar, A., Rastogi, R., Arukonda, S., Shankar, A., Kautish, S., & Sivaram, M. (2020). An efficient hybrid methodology for detection of cancer-causing gene using CSC for micro array data. *Journal of Ambient Intelligence and Humanized Computing*, *11*(11), 4743–4751. doi:10.100712652-020-01731-7

Singh, P., & Dhiman, G. (2017, December). A fuzzy-LP approach in time series forecasting. In *International Conference on Pattern Recognition and Machine Intelligence* (pp. 243-253). Springer. 10.1007/978-3-319-69900-4_31

Singh, P., & Dhiman, G. (2018). A hybrid fuzzy time series forecasting model based on granular computing and bio-inspired optimization approaches. *Journal of Computational Science*, *27*, 370–385. doi:10.1016/j.jocs.2018.05.008

Singh, P., & Dhiman, G. (2018). Uncertainty representation using fuzzy-entropy approach: Special application in remotely sensed high-resolution satellite images (RSHRSIs). *Applied Soft Computing*, *72*, 121–139. doi:10.1016/j.asoc.2018.07.038

Thabtah, F. F. (2017). *Autistic spectrum disorder screening data for children data set.* Academic Press.

Vahia, V. N. (2013). Diagnostic and statistical manual of mental disorders 5: A quick glance. *Indian Journal of Psychiatry*, *55*(3), 220–223. doi:10.4103/0019-5545.117131 PMID:24082241

Voineagu, I., Wang, X., Johnston, P., Lowe, J. K., Tian, Y., Horvath, S., Mill, J., Cantor, R. M., Blencowe, B. J., & Geschwind, D. H. (2011). Transcriptomic analysis of autistic brain reveals convergent molecular pathology. *Nature*, *474*(7351), 380–384. doi:10.1038/nature10110 PMID:21614001

Wang, L. (2017). Datamining, machine learning and big data analytics. *Int. Trans. Electr. Comput. Eng. Syst.*, *4*, 55–61.

Wilhelm-Benartzi, C. S., Koestler, D. C., Karagas, M. R., Flanagan, J. M., Christensen, B. C., Kelsey, K. T., Marsit, C. J., Houseman, E. A., & Brown, R. (2013). Review of processing and analysis methods for DNA methylation array data. *British Journal of Cancer*, *109*(6), 1394–1402. doi:10.1038/bjc.2013.496 PMID:23982603

Winden, K. D., Ebrahimi-Fakhari, D., & Sahin, M. (2018). Abnormal mTOR Activation in Autism. *Annual Review of Neuroscience*, *41*(1), 1–23. doi:10.1146/annurev-neuro-080317-061747 PMID:29490194

Wong, N., Morley, R., Saffery, R., & Craig, J. (2008). Archived Guthrie blood spots as a novel source for quantitative DNA methylation analysis. *Biotechniques, 45*.

Xiao, Z., Qiu, T., Ke, X., Xiao, X., Xiao, T., Liang, F., Zou, B., Huang, H., Fang, H., Chu, K., Zhang, J., & Liu, Y. (2014). Autism spectrum disorder as early neuro developmental disorder: Evidence from the brain imaging abnormalities in 2–3 years old toddlers. *Journal of Autism and Developmental Disorders*, *44*(7), 1633–1640. doi:10.100710803-014-2033-x PMID:24419870

Zwaigenbaum, L., Bauman, M. L., Fein, D., Pierce, K., Buie, T., Davis, P. A., Newschaffer, C., Robins, D. L., Wetherby, A., Choueiri, R., Kasari, C., Stone, W. L., Yirmiya, N., Estes, A., Hansen, R. L., Mc Partland, J. C., Natowicz, M. R., Carter, A., Granpeesheh, D., ... Wagner, S. (2015). Early screening of autism spectrum disorder: Recommendations for practice and research. *Pediatrics*, *136*(Suppl1), S41–S59. doi:10.1542/peds.2014-3667D PMID:26430169

Chapter 3
A Novel Technique on Autism Spectrum Disorders Using Classification Techniques

Jyoti Bhola
National Institute of Technology, Hamirpur, India

Gaurav Dhiman
Government Bikram College of Commerce, Patiala, India

Tarun Singhal
Chandigarh Engineering College, India

Guna Sekhar Sajja
University of the Cumberlands, USA

ABSTRACT

Over the last few years, academic institutions have conducted a number of programmes to help school boards, colleges, and schools of autism spectrum educating pupils (ASD). Autism spectrum disorder (ASD) is a complicated neurological disorder which affects many skills over a lifetime. The main aim of the chapter is to examine the topic of autism and identify autism levels with furious logic classification algorithms using the artificial neural network. Data mining has generally been recognized as a method of decision making to promote higher use of resources for autism students.

DOI: 10.4018/978-1-7998-7460-7.ch003

INTRODUCTION

The ASD is a common neuro develop mentally complex disease. It has a number of combination diseases including intellectual disorders, convulsions and anxiety (Hochberg et. al.,1995). The 2013 study found that 1 of children aged 6-17 years had ASD (Manzardo et. al., 2015). ASDs have moderate to extreme contact and communication impairments and have limited, repeated activity and concerns (Weksberg et. al., 2013). The accuracy of patients with ASD from traditional checks is a critical step (TC). Currently, neuroimaging technology in the treatment of multiple brain conditions, such as ASD, Alzheimer and schizophrenia classification has been extensively used (Vahia, 2013), (Geschwind et. al., 2011).

The self-injurious conduct of children with autism spectrum disorder (ASD) is one of the main sources of hospitalisation (Kalb et al., 2016). The SIB can be repetitive and rhythmic and involve conduct like knockouts and self-hits (Minshawi et al., 2014). SIB can result in physical injury, including abrasions, lacerations and bruising (Rooker et al. 2018), particularly because SIB usually goes past the original age of onset. However, early approaches can help to mitigate serious complications and reduce the continuity of SIB in the long run (Kurtz et al., 2003).

Magnetic resonance imaging (MRI) is a powerful and secure technique that offers high resolution 3D representations of the structure of the brain and accurate structural details. Applied to the associated disorders, morphological experiments on the basis of MRI images obtained successful outcomes. The findings showed that the variable brain and cerebraal heterogeneity are associated with ASD-focused regional cortical thicknesses derived from surface morphologies in order to perform ASD classification and to obtain good classification efficiency (Wange, 2017) using six preselected volume-based features for performing the ASD classification. For example. (Brown et al. 2013) extracted morphologic characteristics for the assessment of Alzheimer's disorder, including mean cortical width, geographic cortical mass etc. (Sahin et. al. 2018) have derived the morphological features of MRI evidence to characterize schizophrenia and have shown that frontal lobe grey matter is below normal controls in schizophrenic patients (Craig et. al.s, 2008).

Autism Spectrum Disorder (ASD) is a polygenetically developing brain disorder with emotional and behavioural mutilation (Liu et. al., 2014). It is a lifetime neurodevelopmental disease that shows speech insufficiencies, interactions and restricted behaviours. Though ASD is primarily characterized through conductal and social physiognomy, autistic persons also have a tainted motor skill, such as lower physical synchronization, unstable body balance and irregular activity and stance (Wagner et. al., 2015). Individuals with ASD exhibit conventional recurring activities, restricted desires, deprivation of mastery of instincts, speech deficiencies, impaired intelligence and cognitive abilities in relation to normal children in development (TD). The diagnosis of ASD using cinematic physiognomies was well known (Abowd et. al., 2012).

However, SIB monitoring requires sophisticated classification methods to detect SIB from dynamic motion data sources, both high performance (i.e. low preparation and classification times), and high precision SIB monitoring (i.e., correctly classified SIB and non-SIB events). Algorithms used often in the detection of human behaviour include supportive vector machines (SVMs), discriminatory analyses (DA), decision trees (DTs), Naïve Bayes (nB), neighbour k-nearest (kNN), and neural networks (NN) (e, for example, (Moreau et al. 2018), (Mittek et al. 2015), (Miller et Al., 2013) etc. In earlier research, movement algorithms were used to identify among ASD-powered persons with up to 89% NN and SVM accuracy when repeat movement was detected. Classification methods previously investigated can extend to the SIB, mainly because previous research has established a connection between SIB and SMMs (Minshawi et al., 2014).

In information analysis, the data mining can be a promising and thriving boundary, and the analysis findings have many applications. Data mining may also be referred to as data discovery (KDD). This method operates as a computer controlled or easy exhaust of trends that indirectly maintain or collect knowledge in huge libraries, data warehouses, the web, data repositories and streams of information. Data mining may be a multidisciplinary field, covering fields such as IT, machine learning, analytics, pattern identification, information processing, artificial neural networks and knowledges, artificial intelligence and data structures. The use of data mining in education systems is widespread. An autism diagnosis is a dynamic cognitive disease, which also impacts the emerging awareness, which can be used to improve understanding of the welfare of autism children, their learning abilities, their coping rates and the achievement rate of Autism students. A central and critical factor for measuring the success of autism students is the data mining system. Classification algorithms are used to correctly and accurately classifying and analyzing student data collection. The key purpose of this paper is to use methods of data mining to research the success of autism students. Data mining offers many activities for studying the success of autism children. The task of this paper is to measure the autism level of students by using the different data mining algorithms of the classification.

Spectrum Autism Disorders Types

The autism spectrum disorders are classified as "parasites," five conditions known as pervasive developing disorders (PDD). They are concerned with the three most popular PDDs, autism, Asperger's syndrome and pertussis-disorder (PDD-NOS)

Some prevalent developmental conditions include childhood disintegration disorder and Rett Syndrome. As each inherited disorder has become extraordinarily rare, it is also considered that each disease does not really belong to the continuum of autism.

Autism Spectrum Disorders Signs and Symptoms

Any kid and adult have problems with social contact, voice and communication in relation to the signs and symptoms of autism spectrum disorders. Autism conditions are measured on the grounds that the child's capacity to talk, to establish relationships, to explore, to play, to study is interrupted by certain symptoms. The individual's approach expresses and concerns individuals. Educational data mining is an emerging field with which education can be successfully implemented. Education data mining employs a number of theories and principles such as the algorithm of the association norm, the grouping algorithm and the algorithm. The signs of autism: social skills. autism disorders. Basic social contact with children with autism spectrum disorders can be troubling. Symptoms may involve unusual or inadequate verbal communication, movements and facial expressions (e.g., avoidance of touch with the eye or of facial phrases that do not complement his or her words).

Lack of concern for individuals or for sharing interests or results (e.g., showing you a drawing, pointing to a bird). It is unlikely that others will approach or attempt social interactions; it seems to be distant and reserved, rather than isolated. Problem and difficulties in interpreting the thoughts, reactions and nonverbal questions of the client. Resistance against being affected. Failure to make friends of children with the same age or difficulty.

Speaking and Language Symptoms in Autism Disorders

Spoken problems and linguistic understanding are a telling symptom of autism spectrum disorders. Speaking in irregular sound of a voice, or in strange rhythms or in high tones could require delay in speech (within age or without minimum talking). Words or expressions repeated time and time again, Problems starting or maintaining a spoken language, Difficulty expressing requirements or wishes, don't see simple sentences or questions, in reality, what is the same, comedy, irony, satire, is absent.

Autism Spectrum Disorders Symptoms: Restricted Conduct and Play

In their behaviour, activities and desires, children with autism specter disorders are often restricted, static and even psycho-neurotic. Repetitive body motion may be symptoms (hand undulation, rocking, spinning). A dark connection to unusual items.

Concern with a specific issue, usually with numbers or symbols (maps, license plates, sports statistics). For sameness, order and rituals, a powerful person wishes. Is disturbed when your schedule or your environment is changed. Slumber, peculiar posture or strange forms to get around. Spinning object, moving objects or toy components are fascinating (e.g., spinning the wheels on a motor car, rather than fidgeting with the whole car). The related autism spectrum disorders signs and symptoms Sensory questions Difficulty emotionally, Uneven psychological characteristic skills.

Autism Support With Children

Autism can be a chronic condition and no remarkable autism treatment is currently available. Besides many autism students, academic efforts in specifically adapted environments will grow considerably with early, well prepared and customized individually (Reyana & Kautish, 2021). The key aims are to help children communicate purposefully. The approaches to education should focus on specific areas in which children with autism learn. Several (Applied behaviour analyses) ABA techniques are examples of these particularly personalized academic interventions for people with autism, as is standardized educational approaches within the (Treatment and Education of Autistic and Related communications Handicapped Children) paradigm. The first is early discovery, diagnosis and evaluation, and the next step is to teach parents proper information (Reyana et al, 2020). The need for child is essential, particularly adapted nursery and subsequent education; a suitable environment of home and even the daily activities of the adults are equally crucial. Adults and young people will continue to access academic initiatives to build skills aimed at expanding.

RELATED WORK

(Wall et. al., 2015) urged that an interactive computer game increase intelligibility via the autistic children's expression. Autism is not definitely handled. To serve autism kids by games and teaching facilities to develop their abilities. In 2013, the Santos explores the first detection of autism, which is to say that using classification techniques controlled SVM, takes the patient signs during adolescence supported by preverbal vocalization (support vector machine). Chaminade, a shot begun in 2012 using MRI for young adults who are autistically engaged with a humanoid robot.

(Langley et. al., 2013) Gesticulation data is used to assess atypical variation in children's facial expressions with and without ASD. Using information theory, mathematical analysis and time series modelling, six face reactions were securitized. Recently, scientists have used data analytics as an ASD diagnostic method to refine and apply them. The possibility for classification in the different domains has been shown to be an effective computer machine learning. Thus, some literature has used machine learning methods to classify neural or behavioural markers which discriminate persons with and without ASD. The power of the eye to identify clusters of children at high or low risk of ASD. Computer techniques were applied, such as the study of discriminating functions of 0.72 precision, 0.69 accuracy vector machine help and 0.89 accuracy linear discriminatory analysis. Bone collected evidence in 2016 from Autism Diagnostical Interview-Revised and Social Responsiveness Scales, and used the SVM machine learning classification for an important person with and without ASD, which produced positive outcomes.

(Wong et. al., 2001) The creation of a predictive model by using a dataset of 32 possible risk elements of pregnancy in autism development was using artificial neural networks (ANN). The predictive accuracy of the artificial neural network is 88 percent. Their research advocated and promoted the use of ANN as an excellent method for the diagnosis of ASD. The best accuracy of classification achieved to date is 96.7% for SVM.

(Radhakrishna et al., 2019) Examines problems in classifying computer training techniques' non-standardized text. It is proposed that ASD may be a terribly heterogeneous condition that will include subgroups with completely different signatures on genetic expression due to the classification issue. To enhance classification, stratification of subgroups of the ASD community and enhance the feedback set by clinical interventions should be beneficial.

(Graham et. al., 2019) Quick Bayesian method for logistical regression used by Laplace before fitting over to prevent sparse text data predictive models. They also used this technique to disperse issues of paper ratings and have shown that they yield lightweight models that are as accurate as compact ones, combined with feature collection, created by vector classification aids or frame logistics regression.

(Abowd et. al., 2012) After three years of clinical observation, surgery and psychiatric therapy the prediction processes (Rani, & Kautish, 2018) were proposed in a group of children with autism. Specifically, psychiatric, developmental, social and demographic approaches were used for the study of children's prognosis with autism. They have tried to predict short-term autism results and classify clinical and personal signs. Initially, data were collected using the Naive Bayes algorithms (Sampathkumar et al, 2020), the General Linear Model, the Logistic Regression and the decision tree from Tracking lists, such as the Autism Checklist, the Aberrant Behavior Control list. Then, the positive or negative results were proportional to the clinical factors frequency. They have chosen to use the decision tree to illustrate the data. This technique allows psychiatrists to find people in sub-groups with autism and other complex disorders in neurodevelopment, even if the results are interim. For grouping purposes, the decision trees are trees. Each tree node represents an immediate element and the product of each branch. Classification laws are described by the roads. It is a fact that facts can be visualized by decision-making bodies.

(Sahin, 2018) Real evidence system for data collection, emulation and auto-stimulation compliance on-the-body accelerometer sensors. According to their initial results on synthetic data, a pathological behaviourally automatic indexing approach was practicable. They use the Marcov Modelle (HMM) to track 7 tunings, including hand-swing and body rocking, from the captured accelerometer. Pathologic behaviour synthetic data is collected about healthy adult neurotypes. Their proposed approach achieves precision rates in a remote and continuous setting.

(Wang, 2017) The proposal for a tracking scheme for generating dictionaries based on characteristics and clustering of statistics on higher order (HOS). In addition, a semi-monitored approach has been used to train the machine in creating models for existing events using a subset of training data to learn about new events. The other part of the testing data has also been used to detect new events in both HOS and LPC. With the previously published findings the proposed algorithm yielded similar results which were based on the supervised method for initial dictionary education. Despite promising accuracy rates, which restrict the use of SMM detection, the process is very difficult.

CLASSIFICATION

This method is used for the classification of data into predefined class labels. A classification procedure consisting of data and test data may be a two-stage process. In the first stage of the study, the data multipliers from training data with the selection of attributes are examined and analyzed. The need for a class mark attribute is known for any tuple of training data. The techniques of classification rules apply to model formation results. The test data was used in the second stage of the classification to check the precision of the model. If the model is suited to its precision, the model can be used to identify unknown tuples of data.

Artificial Neural Network

An ANN consists of a series of linked units or nodes known as artificial neurons that models the neurons loosely in the biological brain. Any relationship can relay a signal to other neurons, such as the synapses of the biological brain. An artificial neuron that receives a signal will then process and signal connected neurons. The signal at the junction is a true number, and a certain non-linear function of the sum of its inputs is the output of each neuron. Figure 1 shows the architecture of ANN.

Figure 1. Artificial Neural Network

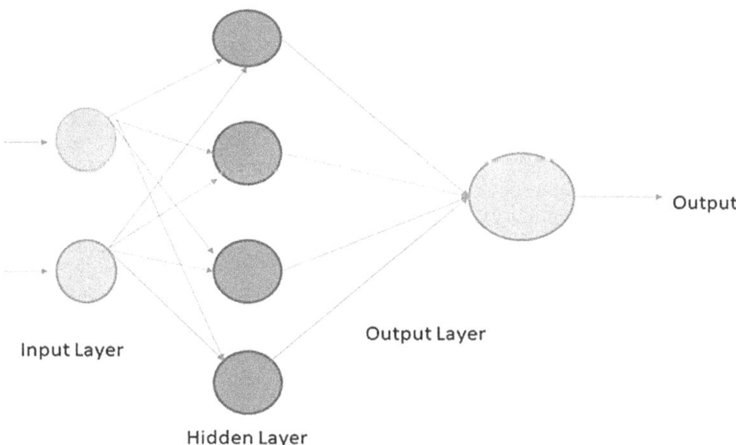

The links are called borders. Usually, neurons and borders are weighty and can be modified through learning. The weight increases or reduces the signal intensity at the links. The threshold of neurons could be where a signal is sent only if the added signal passes beyond the threshold. Neurons are usually combined in layers. Multiple layers can transform their inputs in different ways. Signals move from the first layer (input layer) to the final layer (output layer), presumably following the crossing of the layers many times. The neural artificial network is also usually arranged in layers. Various interconnected 'nodes' that hold a 'activation feature' are used to build layers. Network patterns are provided through the 'input level,' to which one or more 'hidden layers' are transmitted. The secret layers are then connected to an 'output layer.' Most ANNs contain a kind of 'learning law' that changes the connections' weights in accordance to the input patterns.

Fuzzy Logic

In 1965, with the proposal of a 1965 Lotfi A. Zadeh fuszy theory, the term "fuzzy logic" was adopted. Fuzzy logic was extended from the control theory of artificial intelligence in various fields. Fuzzy logic may be a sort of highly valuable logic. Figure 2 shows the schematic layout of the Fuzzy Logic. It deals with thinking approximate, rather than precise, rather than set. Fuzzy logical variables which have a truth that is between 0 and 1 in degrees. The furious logic of part of fact, where Truth Wert will lie in the continuum between absolutely true and totally false, is expanded to deal with it. These degrees are often regulated by special functions until language variables are used.

Figure 2. Fuzzy Logic

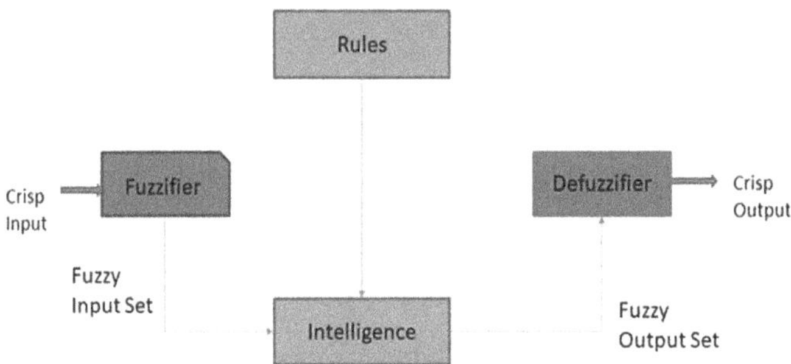

Dataset

Dataset was obtained from the openly available UCI research repository for this report (Thabtah, 2017) (Thabtah et al., 2017); (Murthy, 2001). This research has used autistic data on spectrum condition for infants, data sets and 292 cases and 21 features such as age, ethnicity and nationality of patients. The patient had a Yaundice birth problem, any family member had extensive disability in production, who's done the experiment? The house on which the client resides, previously used screening programme for the user, scanning methods, Multivariate score, reaction based on sampling techniques.

DATA PREPROCESSING

Data sets can be explicit in the classification algorithm and should be preprocessed for managing missing or redundant attributes. In order to maximize data mining operations, the data needs to be processed effectively.

Training and Testing Set

The whole data set was split into two sections, i.e., 70 percent and 30%. One segment is a planning data set, the other section is an analysis data set. The data set collected is shown in Table 1.

Attribute Identification

See Table 1.

Table 1. Dataset collected from autism student database

Parameters	Skills	Values
Language	Speech	Low, Medium, High
Social	Communal	Low, Medium, High
Behavior	Conduct	Low, Medium, High
Extent of ASD	Degree	Low, Medium, High

Results and Discussion

The results are determined with precise and precise accuracy by the Artificial Neural Network. The exact nature of the model depends on the results. Classification research and explanation is a time-consuming task requiring a thorough knowledge of statistics. The models require a lot of time to complete and expert research to examine the classification and relationships in the results. Weka is an open-source software framework which uses a wide range of machine learning algorithms for implementation of the models and is widely used in data mining applications. Autism was developed from the above results. The file has been loaded for a Weka explorer. Different influences, such as speech, emotional, behaviour and autism stages, affect the autism preview of the students. The installation took 400 measurements. The classification panel enables the user to use classification algorithms to the data collection which is applied to evaluate the accuracy of the statistical model of the resulting autism students and to view the model. Weka was assisted by the Neural Network and the Fuzzy logic. The 5-fold-cross validation is selected under the "Test choices." Figure 3 shows the level of Autism.

Figure 3. Level of Autism

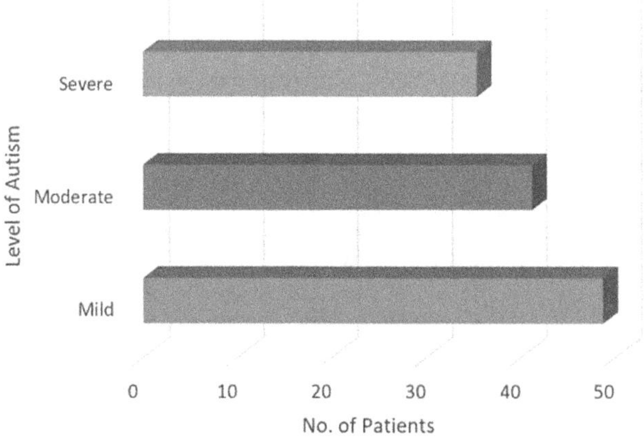

CONCLUSION

Autism spectrum disorders (ASDs) are determined in the presence of restricted attention and repeated conduct, by deficiency of social functioning and expression. Autism should be diagnosed by the behavioral symptoms of all the above areas up to age 3. And if parents usually note that something is wrong in their childhood, autism by the age of 18 months is very difficult to detect. While many children with brain dysfunction and sensory and auditory deficiency are over-represented in this population, many children with autism have a cognitive impairment and behavioral retardation. Persons with autism-like Asperger syndrome have normal or greater intelligence than average. This paper refers to the issue of autism and the different types of autism, and contrasts the efficiency of popular computer education techniques with the fugitive reasoning of the Artificial Neural Network. The findings of this analysis support the development potential of a successful SIB surveillance scheme, which is one of the most dangerous issues in ASD.

REFERENCES

Bahado-Singh, R. O., Vishweswaraiah, S., Aydas, B., Mishra, N. K., Guda, C., & Radhakrishna, U. (2019). Deep learning / artificial intelligence and blood-based DNA epigenomic prediction of cerebralpalsy. *International Journal of Molecular Sciences*, 20. PMID:31035542

Bahado-Singh, R.O., Yilmaz, A., Bisgin, H., Turkoglu, O., Kumar, P., Sherman, E., Mrazik, A., Odibo, A., & Graham, S.F. (2019). Artificial intelligence and the analysis of multiplatform metabolomics data for the detection of intrauterine growth restriction. *PLoS One, 14*.

Bengio, Y. (2009). Learning deep architectures for AI. Found. Trends®. *Machine Learning*, *2*(1), 1–127. doi:10.1561/2200000006

Benjamini, Y., & Hochberg, Y. (1995). Controlling the false discovery rate: A practical and powerful approach to multiple testing. *Journal of the Royal Statistical Society. Series B. Methodological*, *57*(1), 289–300. doi:10.1111/j.2517-6161.1995.tb02031.x

Butler, M. G., Rafi, S. K., Hossain, W., Stephan, D. A., & Manzardo, A. M. (2015). Whole exome sequencing in females with autism implicates novel and candidate genes. *International Journal of Molecular Sciences*, *16*(1), 1312–1335. doi:10.3390/ijms16011312 PMID:25574603

Chen, Y. A., Lemire, M., Choufani, S., Butcher, D. T., Grafodatskaya, D., Zanke, B. W., Gallinger, S., Hudson, T. J., & Weksberg, R. (2013). Discovery of cross-reactive probes and polymorphic CpGs in the Illumina Infinium Human Methylation 450 microarray. *Epigenetics, 8*(2), 203–209. doi:10.4161/epi.23470 PMID:23314698

John, G. H., & Langley, P. (2013). *Estimating continuous distributions in Bayesian classifiers*. arXiv preprint arXiv:1302.4964.

Kaur, R., & Kautish, S. (2019). Multimodal sentiment analysis: A survey and comparison. *International Journal of Service Science, Management, Engineering, and Technology, 10*(2), 38–58. doi:10.4018/IJSSMET.2019040103

Kosmicki, J. A., Sochat, V., Duda, M., & Wall, D. P. (2015). Searching for a minimal set of behaviors for autism detection through feature selection-based machine learning. *Translational Psychiatry, 5*(2), e514–e514. doi:10.1038/tp.2015.7 PMID:25710120

Liu, B., Ma, Y., & Wong, C. K. (2001). Classification using association rules: weaknesses and enhancements. In *Data mining for scientific and engineering applications* (pp. 591–605). Springer. doi:10.1007/978-1-4615-1733-7_30

Plötz, T., Hammerla, N. Y., Rozga, A., Reavis, A., Call, N., & Abowd, G. D. (2012). Automatic assessment of problem behavior in individuals with developmental disabilities. Paper presented at the proceedings of the 2012 ACM conference on ubiquitous computing. 10.1145/2370216.2370276

Plötz, T., Hammerla, N. Y., Rozga, A., Reavis, A., Call, N., & Abowd, G. D. (2012). Automatic assessment of problem behavior in individuals with developmental disabilities. *Proceedings of the 2012 ACM conference on ubiquitous computing*. 10.1145/2370216.2370276

Poliker, R. (2006). Pattern recognition. In *Wiley Encyclopedia of biomedical engineering*. Wiley. doi:10.1002/9780471740360.ebs0904

Poliker, R. (2006). Pattern recognition. In *Wiley Encyclopedia of biomedical engineering*. Wiley. doi:10.1002/9780471740360.ebs0904

Preece, S. J., Goulermas, J. Y., Kenney, L. P., Howard, D., Meijer, K., & Crompton, R. (2009). Activity identification using body-mounted sensors - A review of classification techniques. *Physiological Measurement, 30*(4), R1–R33. doi:10.1088/0967-3334/30/4/R01 PMID:19342767

Rani, S., & Kautish, S. (2018, June). Association clustering and time series based data mining in continuous data for diabetes prediction. In *2018 second international conference on intelligent computing and control systems (ICICCS)* (pp. 1209-1214). IEEE. 10.1109/ICCONS.2018.8662909

Rani, S., & Kautish, S. (2018). Application of data mining techniques for prediction of diabetes-A review. International Journal of Scientific Research in Computer Science. *Engineering and Information Technology*, *3*(3), 1996–2004.

Reyana, A., & Kautish, S. (2021). *Corona virus-related Disease Pandemic: A Review on Machine Learning Approaches and Treatment Trials on Diagnosed Population for Future Clinical Decision Support*. Current Medical Imaging.

Reyana, A., Krishnaprasath, V. T., Kautish, S., Panigrahi, R., & Shaik, M. (2020). Decision-making on the existence of soft exudates in diabetic retinopathy. *International Journal of Computer Applications in Technology*, *64*(4), 375–381. doi:10.1504/IJCAT.2020.112684

Saini, G. K., Chouhan, H., Kori, S., Gupta, A., Shabaz, M., Jagota, V., & Singh, B. K. (2021). Recognition of Human Sentiment from Image using Machine Learning. *Annals of the Romanian Society for Cell Biology*, *25*(5), 1802–1808.

Sampathkumar, A., Rastogi, R., Arukonda, S., Shankar, A., Kautish, S., & Sivaram, M. (2020). An efficient hybrid methodology for detection of cancer-causing gene using CSC for micro array data. *Journal of Ambient Intelligence and Humanized Computing*, *11*(11), 4743–4751. doi:10.100712652-020-01731-7

Singh, P., & Dhiman, G. (2017, December). A fuzzy-LP approach in time series forecasting. In *International Conference on Pattern Recognition and Machine Intelligence* (pp. 243-253). Springer. 10.1007/978-3-319-69900-4_31

Singh, P., & Dhiman, G. (2018). A hybrid fuzzy time series forecasting model based on granular computing and bio-inspired optimization approaches. *Journal of Computational Science*, *27*, 370–385. doi:10.1016/j.jocs.2018.05.008

Singh, P., & Dhiman, G. (2018). Uncertainty representation using fuzzy-entropy approach: Special application in remotely sensed high-resolution satellite images (RSHRSIs). *Applied Soft Computing*, *72*, 121–139. doi:10.1016/j.asoc.2018.07.038

Thabtah, F. F. (2017). *Autistic spectrum disorder screening data for children data set*. Academic Press.

Vahia, V. N. (2013). Diagnostic and statistical manual of mental disorders 5: A quick glance. *Indian Journal of Psychiatry*, *55*(3), 220–223. doi:10.4103/0019-5545.117131 PMID:24082241

Voineagu, I., Wang, X., Johnston, P., Lowe, J. K., Tian, Y., Horvath, S., Mill, J., Cantor, R. M., Blencowe, B. J., & Geschwind, D. H. (2011). Transcriptomic analysis of autistic brain reveals convergent molecular pathology. *Nature*, *474*(7351), 380–384. doi:10.1038/nature10110 PMID:21614001

Wang, L. (2017). Datamining, machine learning and big data analytics. *Int. Trans. Electr. Comput. Eng. Syst., 4*, 55–61.

Wilhelm-Benartzi, C. S., Koestler, D. C., Karagas, M. R., Flanagan, J. M., Christensen, B. C., Kelsey, K. T., Marsit, C. J., Houseman, E. A., & Brown, R. (2013). Review of processing and analysis methods for DNA methylation array data. *British Journal of Cancer, 109*(6), 1394–1402. doi:10.1038/bjc.2013.496 PMID:23982603

Winden, K. D., Ebrahimi-Fakhari, D., & Sahin, M. (2018). Abnormal mTOR Activation in Autism. *Annual Review of Neuroscience, 41*(1), 1–23. doi:10.1146/annurev-neuro-080317-061747 PMID:29490194

Wong, N., Morley, R., Saffery, R., & Craig, J. (2008). Archived Guthrie blood spots as a novel source for quantitative DNA methylation analysis. *Biotechniques, 45.*

Xiao, Z., Qiu, T., Ke, X., Xiao, X., Xiao, T., Liang, F., Zou, B., Huang, H., Fang, H., Chu, K., Zhang, J., & Liu, Y. (2014). Autism spectrum disorder as early neuro developmental disorder: Evidence from the brain imaging abnormalities in 2–3 years old toddlers. *Journal of Autism and Developmental Disorders, 44*(7), 1633–1640. doi:10.100710803-014-2033-x PMID:24419870

Zwaigenbaum, L., Bauman, M. L., Fein, D., Pierce, K., Buie, T., Davis, P. A., Newschaffer, C., Robins, D. L., Wetherby, A., Choueiri, R., Kasari, C., Stone, W. L., Yirmiya, N., Estes, A., Hansen, R. L., Mc Partland, J. C., Natowicz, M. R., Carter, A., Granpeesheh, D., ... Wagner, S. (2015). Early screening of autism spectrum disorder: Recommendations for practice and research. *Pediatrics, 136*(Suppl1), S41–S59. doi:10.1542/peds.2014-3667D PMID:26430169

Chapter 4
A Novel Automated Approach for Deep Learning on Stereotypical Autistic Motor Movements

Mohammad Shabaz
Chitkara University, India

Parveen Singla
Chandigarh Engineering College, India

Malik Mustafa Mohammad Jawarneh
Gulf College, Muscat, Oman

Himayun Mukhtar Qureshi
Birla Institute of Technology and Science, Pilani, India

ABSTRACT

Autism spectrum disorder (ASD) is an ongoing neurodevelopmental disorder, with repeated behavior called stereotypical movement autism (SMM). Some recent experiments with accelerometer features as feedback to computer classifiers demonstrate positive findings in persons with autistic motor disorders for the automobile detection of stereotypical motor motions (SMM). To date, several methods for detecting and recognizing SMMs have been introduced. In this context, the authors suggest an approach of deep learning for recognition of SMM, namely deep convolution neural networks (DCNN). They also implemented a robust DCNN model for the identification of SMM in order to solve stereotypical motor movements (SMM), which thus outperform state-of-the-art SMM classification work.

DOI: 10.4018/978-1-7998-7460-7.ch004

INTRODUCTION

Autism Condition with Continuum ASD refers to a continuum of diseases that can appear at various levels in a number of ways (Association,1994). In social contact, speech and atypical behavior in children with DSA, repetitive behavior is included in children with DSA, motive stereotype children (SMM). Repeat corporal rocking, mouthing, and complicated hand-and-finger gestures are among the most common SMMs (Garmire et. al. 2018), which greatly interfere with learning and social contact while minimizing school and group integration (Graham et. al. 2019), (Sawalha et. al., 2014). Since they are widely immune to psychotropic medications, the purpose of certain therapeutic treatments with autism is to lower or to remove SMMs. And the sooner the age of action, the more your learning and your everyday work will be facilitated (Mori et. al., 2012).

In order to tackle this problem, the role of sensing technology in detecting SMMs during screening and ASD treatment is crucial, which will hopefully improve the lives of people living in the continuum. In fact, it can not only be helpful in finding autistic children but also to consider and intervene on a key symptom of ASD, to diagnose and track SMMs in an efficient and efficient manner over time. SMM must be monitored effectively and reliable as:

- Evaluation of the treatments and/or medicines needed over time and
- Define the mechanisms that cause an SMM such as physiological, emotional or environmental influences. Therapists may use such surveillance to decrease the incidence of SMMs, and their length and intensity progressively (Armstrong, 2008).

The main obstacle to perfect SMM recognition is identified through an automatic function extraction technique from accelerometer signals, using the most critical features that characterizes stereotype behaviours. The heterogeneity in and between subjects (Yilmaz, A) is also a matter of personalization (2018). Due to the changes in magnitude, duration and frequency of MSM in each atypical subject, variances in intra-thirds can also be clarified, while the variances among subjects are due to differences in the amount of MSM in different atypical subjects. An adaptive technique for generalizing and responding to new SMM behaviours is therefore required. With deep SMM learning techniques these issues can be overcome.

We are training two CNN models for detection of SMMs within subjects whose parameters are chosen based on the signal properties of the input SMM. In order to detect the atypical topics in an atypical new field, we are creating a global, fast, lightweight framework for detecting SMM in various fields combining an information transfer mechanism with a classification system for SVMs. One disadvantage of this platform is that very little atypical data from this subject and wide-ranging data from a range of other atypical subjects is labelled in order to address the medical issue of the lack of atypical subject regulated SMMs. Domain-based transmission (i.e., a source region independent from the target domain) provides a suitable SMM recognition quality in an environment on time and adapts the stereotypical enforcement components to every new atypical subject with just a few of the data labels.

Epigenetics means non-mutational genetic modifications. The expression level of the gene is largely influenced by its regulatory regions' epigenetic status. A variety of factors affect gene expression via epigenetic pathways. According to current evidence, epigenetic pathways may play a significant role in ADS production (Hu, 2013) (Loke et al., 2015). The gene MP2 (MECP2), for example, provides an important insight into the potential role of epigenetic pathways for ASD.

Easier, quicker and more objective methods of screening, particularly for younger children, are desperately required to improve those problems. Over the last few decades, a variety of biomarkers have been valued for their ability to recognize people at high risk for ASD development. Such biomarkers evaluate genetic variation, early brain connectivity, perceptual orientation, and other biological processes before the start of the more distinctive behavioral symptoms (Zwaigenbaum and Penner, 2018).

Avoiding an eye or expression of a person is a special pattern of a look in ASD (Fujioka et al., 2016). Measuring ET eye motions has also been widely used in ASD studies, enhancing dramatically our comprehension of gazing habits of the ASD population. Videos or images of individuals are the most commonly used ET paradigm (Annaz et. al., 2012). Studies using this paradigm found gaze abnormalities in ASD people. In these tests, children with ASD had a less time looking at eyes and faces and preferred to stare at insignificant goals than children who were usually developing (TD). These studies (Falck-Ytter et al., 2012). Not only do these results comply with ASD's clinical observations, they also include new information on early diagnosis of ASD. Using metaheuristics (Dhiman & Kumar, 2018), (Dhiman & Kumar, 2018), (Singh & Dhiman, 2018), (Dhiman & Kaur (2017), (Chandrawat et. al, 2017), (Saini et al., 2021), (Singh & Dhiman, 2018), (Dhiman & Kumar, 2019), (Dhiman & Kumar, 2019), (Dhiman & Kaur (2019), (Dhiman & Kumar, 2019), (Singh & Dhiman, 2017), (Kaur & Dhiman 2019), (Dhiman, 2019), (Dhiman, 2019), (Dhiman, 2020), (Dhiman & Kaur, 2019), Dhiman et. al, 2019) researchers are attempted to develop these complex techniques in real life.

The protein binds to methylated DNA regions, while the other gene suppressors bind to the MECP2 and inhibit transcription. In addition, MECP is important for synaptogenesis and long-term synaptic plasticity as it is active in epigenetic regulation of the transcription process throughout the genome (Kavalali et al., 2011). Aberrant

MECP2 (Nagarajan et al. 2006) promoter of methylation is linked to a substantial decrease in the expression of MECP2 protein. Mutations from MECP2 in autism have been identified (Lopez-Rangel & Lewis 2006).

CNN is regarded as a specialist form of neural network that, via back propagation mechanisms, updates weights on any layer of visual hierarchy during training (Radhakrishna et. al., 2019). To have robustness in terms of changes in the input areas and distortions CNN gains from invariant local receptive zones, mutual weights, and spatiotemporal subsampling (Graham et. al., 2019).

The prevalence of prenatal and newborn risk factors in the production of ASD means that newborn screening should be carried out for this condition. Consequently, we investigated the use of DL and other ML strategies for the diagnosis of autism condition (classification system then used during the generation of samples), based on the newborn DNA methylation status. We have also studied the possible epigenetic pathogenesis of autism dependent on cytosine ('CpG' or cg') loci (and associated genes) that have been substantially altered epigenetically.

RELATED WORK

(Bengio, 2009) Proposed manually flopping events using the models of Hidden Markov; however, evidence from stable human imitation behaviors has been obtained. A similar research was carried out, which did not include food for the ADS population (Hochberg et. al., 2015) In the meantime, (Manzardo et.al., 2015), reports were obtained from the wrists and torso of four people with autism for a total of 40 hours of three-axle acceleration results. They obtained high accuracy rates of 82 per cent with hand flap and 97 per cent with respect to corporal rocking, however, with a rarity of various features and semi–supervised classification approaches (orthogonal flap, liner predictive coding, all pole autoregressive model, higher order statistics, ordinary lower positions, K-VSD algorithm).

(Weksberg et. al., 2013) suggested data obtained from the handles and torso of six adults with autism, three axis acceleration, is used regularly in both laboratories and school environments. Through integrating time and frequency-domain characteristics (distance between medium values along axis accelerometers, variation along axis directions, coefficient of correlation, entropy, Fast Fourier Transformation (FFT) peaks and the transformation of Stocks well) to C4.5, SVM and DT classifiers, the overall accuracy of the SMM detection can be achieved.

(Vahia, 2013) In order to obtain much greater accuracy than that, Goodwin has now introduced a proposed new set of characteristics that draw on repeat tracks and analysis quantification, along with decision trees and random forest classifiers.

(Geschwind et. al., 2011) to detect only one kind of SMM, namely flattening manually, use the Kinect (Microsoft) webcam sensor. But the Kinect sensor tracks and helps the users to be close to the sensor within a confined space.

(Sahin, 2018) proposed the proof-of-concept framework for on-the-body accelerometer sensors data acquisition, simulation, and self-stimulatory behaviours. According to their preliminary findings on synthetic evidence, an automated indexation method was feasible for pathological behaviours. They used the Marcov-model (HMM) to detect seven tunings from the captured accelerometer, including hand-swinging and body rocking. Synthetic evidence on stable adult neurotypes emulate pathological behavior are gathered. In the isolated and continuous environment, their proposed method achieves accuracy rates.

(Wang, 2017) proposed the monitoring atoms dictionary generation system based on the characteristics and clustering of the Higher Order Statistics (HOS). In addition, in order to learn new events, a semi-supervised method was used to train the system to generate models for known events using a sub-pack of training data. The other portion of the training data was also used to uncheck the HOS and LPC for new incidents. The proposed algorithm yielded comparable results, which were based on the controlled approach for initial dictionary education, with the previously published results. The process has high difficulty, despite promising precision speeds, which limits the use of SMM detection.

(Gowen et. al.,2017) proposed the way to understand whether SMMs can be correctly identified on the new data set by the qualified classificatory on the old dataset. The authors have wanted to test the strength of a generalized SMM detector from a range of topics to a new topic. Stock well transforms features have been derived from the collected data with five times and frequency domain features, close to the previous analysis. However, the experimental findings in multiple topics indicated a high heterogeneity. It is concluded that the development of adaptive algorithms which spread through subjects and over long interval periods is an urgent need for SMM detection in real-time scenarios, which must be accurate and reliable.

ASD DETECTION METHOD

In this paper, we assume that deep convolutionary neural networks (DCNN) provide more precise SMM sensors and a more robust platform for the learning of inertial signals, thereby enabling this knowledge of representation to be effective and a new dataset, that is crucial in longitudinal studies. In this paper we are assuming that (Langley et. al., 2013). Features including the time-domain and the frequency-domain functions are commonly used for the accelerometer signal operation detection as shown in table1.

ASD data set consists of time series data which consist of measurements on multiple sensor devices on multiple channels M, i.e., x, y, and z. The first step is to transform these M-channel raw data into several fixed length signals, which are referred to as frames, for both the time field and the frequency fields. The next step is to normalize the frames until they are fed to our profound education system.

Deep Convolutionary Neural Networks (DCNNs) take advantage of invariant local receptive fields, common weights and space-time sub-sampling features in order to provide robustness over input change and distortion. DCNN has a hierarchical architecture which alternates convolutionary and bundled layers to synthesize broad intrusion areas with space/time relationships into a smaller dimension. A single dimensional layer is made up of filters, i.e., receptive areas:

$$\phi = \left[F_j^i \in R^f \mid j \in \{1,2,3,\ldots\ldots,F\}\} \right] \quad (1)$$

Where f represents the size of filter, R represents the activation function, which learn different patterns on a time window of time-series. In reality, these filters are to be learnt from the input data. With the input signal through canals each filter is sequentially converted. The output is then transferred to the operator by an activation function to calculate the functional maps $M \in R^{n\times f\times d}$. A linear unit (ReLU) is typically employee of a profound architecture with ReLU(a) = maximum {0, a}, as a function to enable. The characteristic maps are supplied to an additional layer, known as the pooling layer, which conducts local averages or subsampling to reduce the sensitivity of the outcomes to changes and distortions. In fact, a pooling layer reduces the resolution of a feature map by factor of $\frac{1}{k}$, where k is the stride size. Two widely used pooling functions that calculate maximum or average value in the pooling window are the Max and Average pooling systems. This aggregation is done separately within each characteristic map and provides $I \in R^{n\times f\times d/k}$ as the output of pooling layer. As an input in a multi-layer architecture I can be used for another convolutionary i+1 layer. Figure 1 shows 1-dimensional deep layers of convolution.

Figure 1. Architecture of DCNN

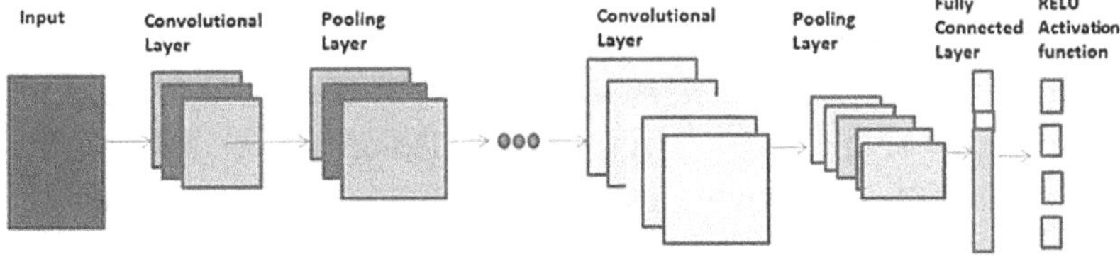

In the following, we suggest the use of a five-layer DCNN to convert multi-accelerometer sensors into a new space for the time series. The pull-out window duration and the bottom line are set to w = 5. The 5-pool phase decreases the length of the characteristic maps after each pooling operation by factor 0.5. The contribution of the fifth cooler layer provides the acquired vector after flattening. To anticipate names, the function vector is fed into a classification. It can be deployed inside the current deep learning technologies.

Since ASD is dynamic, heterogeneous and chronogeny, clinical guidelines typically advise multidisciplinary teams that participate in ASD diagnosis. The Autism Diagnostic Observation Scheme (ADOS) and the Revised Autism Diagnostic Interview (ADI-R) have the greatest sensitivity and specificities of the different diagnostic devices available. While these methods can recognize patterns linked to ASD, many consumers have noticed problems with "diagnostic prejudice and services available." In particular, the use of ADOS and ADI-R continues to include significant time costs and can result in over-diagnosis of ASD.

Since each data instance has D channels, each channel has to be independently normalised. A channel-specific standardisation is achieved to scale all [-1 1] values in the following formula:

$$x_n = (x - x) / \sigma \tag{2}$$

where the data in the particular channel is xn, the mean is x, n means normalization, and σ its standard deviation.

Multiple hyperparameters should be carefully selected in deep neural networks (DCNN) to optimize the efficiency of the network and to obtain the best grading rate. Two types of hyperparameters are available:

- Approximate optimization hyperparameters such as the learning rate, momentum, scale of the minibatch and number of iterations of training

The model hyperparameters and training conditions, such as number of hidden layers, scale (i.e., number of maps) of the layers, the filter size and the regularization (dropout).

One of the parameters to be determined is the filter size of the first congestion layer of the DCNN. In reality, the right first layer filter selection generates pictures informing the input signal and capturing the best fluctuations of the input signal. A small filter is a part of a signal peak only, and thus no maximum fluctuation is detected inside the signal. The big filter is rounded up at the same time by 2 or 3 signal peaks. The filter's optimum size is a signal summit whole. It is then necessary to determine the optimal time for all signal peaks within the input signal. In order to provide statistical details on the population as a whole, we use the sampling process - a statistical technique that involves collecting certain measurements. We use inferential statistics for approximating population characteristics the sample features (i.e., the maximum sample size derived from the random signal selected) (i.e., the optimal peak length of all signals). Survey figures may be average, medium or fashionable. In our study, we either prefer:

- The sample mean or
- A median (statistical) survey for calculating mean and median population, respectively.

We concentrate in our research on DCNN hyperparameters, the DCNN architecture. Generally, the construction of DCNN's architecture is not a common concept. In fact, the testing and error procedure is applied for such criteria, such as the number of function maps, under which many tests are performed by variable values and the ideal value is that which provides the best classification rate. Other parameters, such as the properties of the variations within the input signals, can be determined based on their original input configuration, such as the filter size and the number of layers hidden.

RESULTS AND DISCUSSIONS

The assessment is carried out by F1 calculations. In terms of classification on the raw data, the higher classification performances obtained by the learning features demonstrate the significance of function extraction for SMM prediction. The Comparison of Goodwin et al' and CNN/transferred-findings CNN's shows the effectiveness of the manual functional acquisition features in the SMM forecast. Our result shows finally that the transfer of information between datasets will increase the classification efficiency in longitudinal studies by pre-initializing CNN.

It is to develop the optimal value of the hyperparameters of the CNN model. The feedback of the data used in the "SMM" studies. As discussed in the methodology some parameters such as the size of a function map are defined by trial and error, while others are calculated based on the initial configuration of the input, such as the filter size of convolutionary layers and a number of cached layers. In these dimensions we then evaluate the discrepancy in the CNN performance. F1 results in substantial improvements from 75.04 to 95.87% for the CNN time domain and slightly from 96.04 to 97.00% for the CNN frequency domain. This means that the CNN time domain needs more function cards for capturing both low and medium-level features of the input speed indicators compared to the frequency domain CNN.

Table 1. F1-score for time-domain and frequency-domain

F-Score	20-40	40-60	60-80	80-100	100-120	120-140
Time Domain	62	67	75	87	96	97
Frequency Domain	85	87	88	88	90	92

Because of the high dropout rate, a sufficiently large number of layers is particularly necessary to select. Given the small size of the inputs and the kernel dimension of the first cooling layer, the number of layers stackable at frequency is 5, 3 cooling and sub-sample layers, and 2 completely connected layers and 4, 4 cooling and subsampling layers and 3 fully connected layers, as seen in Figure 2 shows that inputs are of low volume. The objective of the experiment is to explore the relationship between distinct and related characteristics of an atypical subject. First, we assume that the characteristic elements at high levels vary and are responsible for these differences, depending on an atypical theme. We want to see if these atypical subjects share the low and medium levels that the CNN learned in time and frequency.

Figure 2 shows SMM classification for time and frequency. In real-life, in the medical diagnosis of the autism condition, few cases of SMM are available, and computing tools include a light-sized general SMM detection system, which detects SMMs from a new topic based on a limited number of cases of its SMM.

With a mean time and frequency score of 76.42% and 83.02%, this method delivers satisfied results. It thus seems satisfactory to create low- and mid-level functionalities with the characteristics of basic movements and the modification

Figure 2. SMM classification for the time and frequency-domain

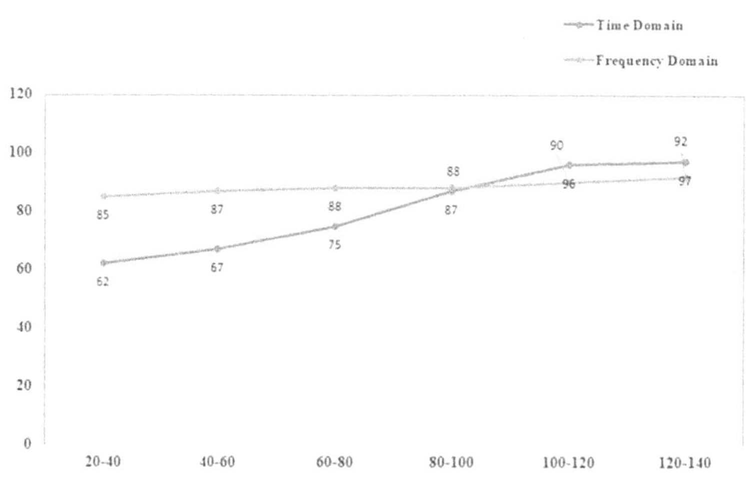

by SVM of only high-level functions and this confirmation of the stereotypical signals of movement detectors used by our method. These results, particularly the frequency domain results.

The low and mid-level properties of basic movements and certain high-level functions, as learned from an Atypically Subject data set from the SVM, is significant, suggesting that humans and stereotypes may share similar low- and mid-level characteristics.

The assessment is carried out by calculating F1 ratings, due to extremely unbalanced grades. The bar diagrams reflect the F1 mark of four separate Study1 and Study2 processes. The x-axis is the ID and mean outcomes on all subjects (M). The outcomes of studies are deterministic on the one-topic abandonment situation on the first and second experiments. Consequently, there is no error record. An analysis of the cumulative output of two datasets reveals the following initial results:

- The improved DCNN classification results and the learned features in comparison to the raw data classification highlight the importance of feature extraction/learning to forecast SMM.
- Findings DCNN's shows the effectiveness of the manual functional acquisition features in the SMM forecast.
- Our result shows finally that the transfer of information between datasets will increase the classification efficiency in longitudinal studies by reinitializing CNN.

CONCLUSION

In this research, we suggested an implementation of profound SMM prediction learning for accelerometer-used ASD infants. Our theoretical studies have shown that the DCNN approaches the conventional handcrafted definition of the deeper neural network. This discovery confirms our initial hypothesis that deep neural networks can train and move more reliable SMM sensing systems. The study shows us the feasibility of embedded functionality learning. This thesis is an early attempt to improve SMM detectors in real time. A device like this can be built into a smartphone application for the omnipresent identification of SMM. The enhanced outcomes of DCNN classification and the learned features in relation to the raw data classification illustrate the importance of SMM feature removal/learning.

REFERENCES

Alakwaa, F. M., Chaudhary, K., & Garmire, L. X. (2018). Deep learning accurately predicts estrogen receptor status in breast cancer metabolomics data. *Journal of Proteome Research*, *17*(1), 337–347. doi:10.1021/acs.jproteome.7b00595 PMID:29110491

Alpay Savasan, Z., Yilmaz, A., Ugur, Z., Aydas, B., Bahado Singh, R. O., & Graham, S. F. (2019). Metabolomic profiling of cerebral palsy brain tissue reveals nove lcentral biomarkers and biochemical path ways associated with the disease: A pilot study. *Metabolites*, 9. PMID:30717353

Altorok, N., Tsou, P. S., Coit, P., Khanna, D., & Sawalha, A. H. (2014). *Genomewide DNA methylation analysis in dermal fibroblasts from patients with diffuse and limited systemic sclerosis reveals common and subset specific DNA methylation aberrancies. In Diagnostic and Statistical Manual of Mental Disorders (5th ed.).* American Psychiatric Association.

Anitha, A., Nakamura, K., Thanseem, I., Yamada, K., Iwayama, Y., Toyota, T., Matsuzaki, H., Miyachi, T., Yamada, S., Tsujii, M., Tsuchiya, K. J., Matsumoto, K., Iwata, Y., Suzuki, K., Ichikawa, H., Sugiyama, T., Yoshikawa, T., & Mori, N. (2012). Brain region -specific altered expression and association of mitochondria related genesinautism. *Molecular Autism*, *3*(1), 12. doi:10.1186/2040-2392-3-12 PMID:23116158

Armstrong, C. (2008). AA Preleases guidelines on identification of children with autism spectrum disorders. *American Family Physician*, *78*, 1301–1305.

Association, A. P. (1994). Diagnostic and Statistical Manual of Mental Disorders (4th ed.). Washington, DC: Author.

Bahado-Singh, R. O., Sonek, J., McKenna, D., Cool, D., Aydas, B., Turkoglu, O., Bjorndahl, T., Mandal, R., Wishart, D., Friedman, P., Graham, S. F., & Yilmaz, A. (2018). Artificial Intelligence and amniotic fluid multiomics analysis: The prediction of perinatal outcome in a symptomatic short cervix. *Ultrasound in Obstetrics & Gynecology*.

Bahado-Singh, R. O., Vishweswaraiah, S., Aydas, B., Mishra, N. K., Guda, C., & Radhakrishna, U. (2019). Deep learning / artificial intelligence and blood-based DNA epigenomic prediction of cerebralpalsy. *International Journal of Molecular Sciences*, 20. PMID:31035542

Bahado-Singh, R.O., Yilmaz, A., Bisgin, H., Turkoglu, O., Kumar, P., Sherman, E., Mrazik, A., Odibo, A., & Graham, S.F., (2019). Artificial intelligence and the analysis of multi-platform metabolomics data for the detection of intrauterine growth restriction. *PLoS One, 14*.

Bengio, Y. (2009). Learning deep architectures for AI. Found. Trends ®, *Machine Learning*, *2*(1), 1–127. doi:10.1561/2200000006

Benjamini, Y., & Hochberg, Y. (1995). Controlling the false discovery rate: A practical and powerful approach to multiple testing. *Journal of the Royal Statistical Society. Series B. Methodological*, *57*(1), 289–300. doi:10.1111/j.2517-6161.1995.tb02031.x

Butler, M. G., Rafi, S. K., Hossain, W., Stephan, D. A., & Manzardo, A. M. (2015). Whole exome sequencing in females with autism implicates novel and candidate genes. *International Journal of Molecular Sciences*, *16*(1), 1312–1335. doi:10.3390/ijms16011312 PMID:25574603

Chen, Y. A., Lemire, M., Choufani, S., Butcher, D. T., Grafodatskaya, D., Zanke, B. W., Gallinger, S., Hudson, T. J., & Weksberg, R. (2013). Discovery of cross-reactive probes and polymorphic CpGs in the Illumina Infinium Human Methylation 450 microarray. *Epigenetics*, *8*(2), 203–209. doi:10.4161/epi.23470 PMID:23314698

Dhiman, G. (2019a). ESA: A hybrid bio-inspired metaheuristic optimization approach for engineering problems. *Engineering with Computers*, 1–31. doi:10.100700366-019-00826-w

Dhiman, G. (2019b). *Multi-objective Metaheuristic Approaches for Data Clustering in Engineering Application (s)* (Doctoral dissertation).

Dhiman, G. (2020). MOSHEPO: A hybrid multi-objective approach to solve economic load dispatch and micro grid problems. *Applied Intelligence*, *50*(1), 119–137. doi:10.100710489-019-01522-4

Dhiman, G., & Kaur, A. (2017, December). Spotted hyena optimizer for solving engineering design problems. In *2017 international conference on machine learning and data science (MLDS)* (pp. 114-119). IEEE.

Dhiman, G., & Kaur, A. (2018). Optimizing the design of air foil and optical buffer problems using spotted hyena optimizer. *Designs*, *2*(3), 28. doi:10.3390/designs2030028

Dhiman, G., & Kaur, A. (2019). A hybrid algorithm based on particle swarm and spotted hyena optimizer for global optimization. In *Soft Computing for Problem Solving* (pp. 599–615). Springer. doi:10.1007/978-981-13-1592-3_47

Dhiman, G., & Kaur, A. (2019). STOA: A bio-inspired based optimization algorithm for industrial engineering problems. *Engineering Applications of Artificial Intelligence*, *82*, 148–174. doi:10.1016/j.engappai.2019.03.021

Dhiman, G., & Kumar, V. (2017). Spotted hyena optimizer: A novel bio-inspired based metaheuristic technique for engineering applications. *Advances in Engineering Software*, *114*, 48–70. doi:10.1016/j.advengsoft.2017.05.014

Dhiman, G., & Kumar, V. (2018). Emperor penguin optimizer: A bio-inspired algorithm for engineering problems. *Knowledge-Based Systems*, *159*, 20–50. doi:10.1016/j.knosys.2018.06.001

Dhiman, G., & Kumar, V. (2018). Multi-objective spotted hyena optimizer: A multi-objective optimization algorithm for engineering problems. *Knowledge-Based Systems*, *150*, 175–197. doi:10.1016/j.knosys.2018.03.011

Dhiman, G., & Kumar, V. (2019). KnRVEA: A hybrid evolutionary algorithm based on knee points and reference vector adaptation strategies for many-objective optimization. *Applied Intelligence*, *49*(7), 2434–2460. doi:10.100710489-018-1365-1

Dhiman, G., & Kumar, V. (2019). Seagull optimization algorithm: Theory and its applications for large-scale industrial engineering problems. *Knowledge-Based Systems*, *165*, 169–196. doi:10.1016/j.knosys.2018.11.024

Dhiman, G., & Kumar, V. (2019). Spotted hyena optimizer for solving complex and non-linear constrained engineering problems. In *Harmony search and nature inspired optimization algorithms* (pp. 857–867). Springer. doi:10.1007/978-981-13-0761-4_81

John, G. H., & Langley, P. (2013). *Estimating continuous distributions in Bayesian classifiers*. arXiv preprint arXiv:1302.4964.

Li, B., Sharma, A., Meng, J., Purushwalkam, S., & Gowen, E. (2017). Applying machine learning to identify autistic adults using imitation: An exploratory study. *PLoS One*, *12*(8), e0182652. doi:10.1371/journal.pone.0182652 PMID:28813454

Plötz, T., Hammerla, N. Y., Rozga, A., Reavis, A., Call, N., & Abowd, G. D. (2012). Automatic assessment of problem behavior in individuals with developmental disabilities. *Proceedings of the 2012 ACM conference on ubiquitous computing*. 10.1145/2370216.2370276

Poliker, R. (2006). Pattern recognition. In *Wiley Encyclopaedia of biomedical engineering*. Wiley. doi:10.1002/9780471740360.ebs0904

Preece, S. J., Goulermas, J. Y., Kenney, L. P., Howard, D., Meijer, K., & Crompton, R. (2009). Activity identification using body-mounted sensors-A review of classification techniques. *Physiological Measurement, 30*(4), R1–R33. doi:10.1088/0967-3334/30/4/R01 PMID:19342767

Pugliese, C. E., Kenworthy, L., Bal, V. H., Wallace, G. L., Yerys, B.E., & Maddox, B. B. (2015). Replication and comparison of the newly proposed ADOS-2, module 4 algorithm in ASD with-out ID: A multi-site study. *Journal of Autism and Developmental Disorders, 45*(12), 3919–3931. . doi:10.100710803-015-2586-3

Saini, G. K., Chouhan, H., Kori, S., Gupta, A., Shabaz, M., Jagota, V., & Singh, B. K. (2021). Recognition of Human Sentiment from Image using Machine Learning. *Annals of the Romanian Society for Cell Biology, 25*(5), 1802–1808.

Singh, P., & Dhiman, G. (2017, December). A fuzzy-LP approach in time series forecasting. In *International Conference on Pattern Recognition and Machine Intelligence* (pp. 243-253). Springer. 10.1007/978-3-319-69900-4_31

Singh, P., & Dhiman, G. (2018). A hybrid fuzzy time series forecasting model based on granular computing and bio-inspired optimization approaches. *Journal of Computational Science, 27*, 370–385. doi:10.1016/j.jocs.2018.05.008

Singh, P., & Dhiman, G. (2018). Uncertainty representation using fuzzy-entropy approach: Special application in remotely sensed high-resolution satellite images (RSHRSIs). *Applied Soft Computing, 72*, 121–139. doi:10.1016/j.asoc.2018.07.038

Vahia, V. N. (2013). Diagnostic and statistical manual of mental disorders 5: A quick glance. *Indian Journal of Psychiatry, 55*(3), 220–223. doi:10.4103/0019-5545.117131 PMID:24082241

Voineagu, I., Wang, X., Johnston, P., Lowe, J.K., Tian, Y., Horvath, S., Mill, J., Cantor, R.M., Blencowe, B.J., & Geschwind, D.H. (2011). Transcriptomic analysis of autistic brain reveals convergent molecular pathology. *Nature, 474*, 380–384.

Wang, L. (2017). Datamining, machine learning and big data analytics. *Int. Trans. Electr. Comput. Eng. Syst., 4*, 55–61.

Wilhelm-Benartzi, C. S., Koestler, D. C., Karagas, M. R., Flanagan, J. M., Christensen, B. C., Kelsey, K. T., Marsit, C. J., Houseman, E. A., & Brown, R. (2013). Review of processing and analysis methods for DNA methylation array data. *British Journal of Cancer, 109*(6), 1394–1402. doi:10.1038/bjc.2013.496 PMID:23982603

Winden, K. D., Ebrahimi-Fakhari, D., & Sahin, M. (2018). Abnormal mTOR Activation in Autism. *Annual Review of Neuroscience, 41*(1), 1–23. doi:10.1146/annurev-neuro-080317-061747 PMID:29490194

Wong, N., Morley, R., Saffery, R., & Craig, J. (2008). Archived Guthrie blood spots as a novel source for quantitative DNA methylation analysis. *Biotechniques, 45*.

Xiao, Z., Qiu, T., Ke, X., Xiao, X., Xiao, T., Liang, F., Zou, B., Huang, H., Fang, H., Chu, K., Zhang, J., & Liu, Y. (2014). Autism spectrum disorder as early neuro developmental disorder: Evidence from the brain imaging abnormalities in 2–3 years old toddlers. *Journal of Autism and Developmental Disorders*, *44*(7), 1633–1640. doi:10.100710803-014-2033-x PMID:24419870

Zwaigenbaum, L., Bauman, M. L., Fein, D., Pierce, K., Buie, T., Davis, P. A., Newschaffer, C., Robins, D. L., Wetherby, A., Choueiri, R., Kasari, C., Stone, W. L., Yirmiya, N., Estes, A., Hansen, R. L., McPartland, J. C., Natowicz, M. R., Carter, A., Granpeesheh, D., ... Wagner, S. (2015). Early screening of autism spectrum disorder: Recommendations for practice and research. *Pediatrics*, *136*(Suppl1), S41–S59. doi:10.1542/peds.2014-3667D PMID:26430169

Chapter 5
Machine Learning Techniques for Analysing and Identifying Autism Spectrum Disorder

Jyoti Bhola
National Institute of Technology, Hamirpur, India

Rubal Jeet
Chandigarh Engineering College, India

Malik Mustafa Mohammad Jawarneh
Gulf College, Muscat, Oman

Shadab Adam Pattekari
https://orcid.org/0000-0002-5231-7216
Indala Group of Institutions, Kalyan, India

ABSTRACT

Autism spectrum disorder (ASD) is a neuro disorder in which a person's contact and connection with others has a lifetime impact. In all levels of development, autism can be diagnosed as a "behavioural condition," since signs generally occur within the first two years of life. The ASD problem begins with puberty and goes on in adolescence and adulthood. In this chapter, an effort is being made to use the supporting vector machine (SVM) and the convolutionary neural network (CNN) for prediction and interpretation of children's ASD problems based on the increased use of machine learning methodology in the research dimension of medical diagnostics. On freely accessible autistic spectrum disorder screening dates in children's datasets, the suggested approaches are tested. Using different techniques of machine learning, the findings clearly conclude that CNN-based prediction models perform more precisely on the dataset for autistic spectrum disorders.

DOI: 10.4018/978-1-7998-7460-7.ch005

INTRODUCTION

The autism spectrum disorder (ASD) epidemic has evolved steadily in all human age groups today. Early diagnosis of this neurological disorder will help significantly to preserve the mental and physical health of the subject. The early identification based on different health and physiological parameters now seems to have become feasible as machine learning model implementations in the predictions of various humans' diseases are increased. This has prompted us to expand our interest in ASD disease diagnosis and analysis in order to develop the technique for treatment. Detecting ASD would be a difficulty, since there are many other psychiatric conditions, the few with ASD manifestations somewhat similar, making this job impossible (Maddox et. al., 2015).

Neuropsychiatric conditions represent 14% of the worldwide illness burden and are the world's leading source of injury related to non-communicable diseases (Axelrod et. al.,1999). The Autism Spectrum Disorder (ASD), which has increased prevalence by around 700 per cent since 1996 and now has an effect 1 in 59 children in the United States, contributes significantly to this metric. As supporting a child with a disease costs up to $2.4 million over their lifetime and health insurance costs ASD probably constitutes one of the biggest paediatric health challenges (Kessler et. al., 2016).

Autism Disorder is an issue that is linked to the growth of the human brain. An Autism Spectrum Disorder sufferer is usually unable to communicate with others socially (Thabtah et. al., 2019), (Rajab et al., 2018), (Sasikala et. al., 2018). This typically influences a person's life throughout his/her life. It is interesting to note that the causative factors for this condition can be both environmental and genetic factors. The symptoms of this issue will begin at the age of three and continue throughout life (Crompton et. al.,2009). The patient with this condition cannot be finished, although the results will be minimized for a limited duration if the signs are identified early in the day. The precise causes of ASD have not yet been recognized by the doctor, believing that human genes are responsible for it. Human genes influence growth through environmental influences. There's a risk factor that affects ASD, such as a low birth weight, an ASD sibler and elderly parents. Instead, some social experiences and contact difficulties occur (McCosh et. al.,1986), such as:

- No pain perception
- Incapable of making good eye contact
- No correct sound answer
- Do not want to be cuddled
- No engagement with others
- Inadequate attachments

- Want to live alone
- Use of echo terms
- No connection with other items

While autism spectrum disorders (ASD) have been regarded as neural in nature, brain biomarkers are uncertain and diagnoses are mostly dependent on behavioral guidelines (Sampathkumar et al, 2020). For this purpose the Autism Brain Imaging Data Exchange (EBIS), selected 252 lowmotion resting-state (LMRI) scans, including TD and ASD usually (n= 126), that corresponded to the non-verbal IQ, head motion and age.People with ASD can sometimes trouble with restricted desires and behavior. In this list you will find particular instances of behavior styles.

- Repeat such habits such as repeating phrases or sentences a great deal of time.
- When a pattern shifts, the individual will be frustrated.
- Have a small interest in certain issues, such as figures, facts, etc.
- In some situations, less sensitive than anyone else such as light, noise, etc.

Early diagnosis and therapy are the key measures to reduce the effects of autism disease and to increase the quality of life of ASD patients. Yet there is no medical screening protocol for autism diagnosis. Symptoms of ASD usually seen by observation (Olivier et. al.,2011). ASD signs are usually detected by the parents and the teachers of older adults and teenagers who go to kindergarten. A special school education committee examines the symptoms of ASD afterwards. These school teams recommended that these children consult their doctor for appropriate exams (Narayanan et. al.,2014), (Abowd et. al., 2012). Adults are harder to recognize ASD symptoms than older kids and young people since those ASD symptoms may correlate with other mental health conditions. The behavioural differences in children may easily be detected by examination, since autism-specific brain imaging can be seen earlier in the 6 months, as brain scans may be noticeable after 2 years of age (DeLuca et. al., 2012).

LITERATURE SURVEY

(Sasikala et. al. 2018) proposed a tool to define optimum behaviour sets for Autism. In this paper a DSA dataset with 21 functions from the UCI learning depot experimented with a binary firefly collection wrapper focused on swarm intelligence. The alternative hypothesis of the experiment says that a machine learning algorithm can be accomplished with minimal feature subsets for greater classification precision. It is observed that ten functions of 21 features of the ASD dataset are adequate to differentiate between patients with ASD and non-ASD by using the single-target. The findings achieved in this method justify the idea that an average accuracy of 92,12% - 97,95% for optimum function subsets is roughly equivalent to the ASD diagnostic data collection. The results of this approach show that they are approximating the average accuracy.

(Thabtah et. al., 2017) also suggested a Machine Learning model of the ASD. One or more ASD screening targets is realized with a screening tool. This essay addressed the ASD classification of machine learning with their benefits and drawbacks. Instead of the DSM-5 manual, the researcher has sought to illustrate the issue with current ASD screening methods and the accuracy of those tools.

(Shanavas et. al., 2014) proposed a Classification Strategies ASD analysis. The primary objective of this paper was the identification of autism and autism stages. SVM and Fuzzy methods are used in this Neural Network with WEKA software to analyze the behavior of students and their social experiences.

(Wall et. al., 2015) supposed a framework for looking for a minimal range of characteristics for diagnosis of autism. The investigators used an automated approach to research ASD's clinical examination. The ADOS was conducted on the basis of the autism spectrum of children's behavior. Eight various machine-learning algorithms have been used to gradually identify features from 4,540 entities, on score sheets. The ASD vulnerability detecting an average precision of 98.27 percent and 97.66% of 28 activities in module 2 and 12 from module 3 detects a risk of ASD.

(Abowd et. al., 2012) proposed the prediction mechanisms were tested in a population of children with autism after 3-year clinical observation, operation and psychiatric treatment. Mechanical methods for the study of psychiatric, developmental, social and demographic aspects, which influence child prognosis with autism, were used specifically. They also attempted to forecast short-term autism outcomes and to identify health and personal causes affecting the symptoms.Initially, data were obtained from monitoring lists such as the Checklist for Autism and the Aberrant Behavior Checklist and evaluated using the Naïve Bayes algorithms, the Generalized linear model, the Logistic Regression and the Decision Tree. They then correlated the positive or bad effects to the frequency of the clinical variables. To explain the data, they decided to use the decision tree. This approach will allow psychiatric doctors to detect patients in autism sub groups and other complicated neuro-development conditions, even though the findings are provisional.Decision trees are trees for classification purposes. Every tree node represents an immediate element and every branch represents the result. The combined paths represent the laws of classification. It is a reality that information can be visualized by means of decision-making trees.

(Gowen et. al., 2017) machine learning classifiers are used to imitate autistic people. The objective of this thesis was to study the underlying issue of discriminatory test conditions and cinematic criteria. The dataset includes 16 ASC participants with a number of hand gestures. The use of machine learning techniques eliminated 40 cinematics restrictions from 08 imitation conditions. This study reveals that a small sample can be used to analyses high-dimensional data and autism diagnosis recognition through machine learning approaches.

The potential for the implementation of profound learning models for ASD identification in people from the above section is obviously important to review. Most of the above work uses conventional machine training techniques and thereby reduces their performance. The results of several Master Learning models (Rani & Kautish, 2018) were compared to the profound learning model. Separate models were developed and compared separately with a diverse demographic set.

DATASET

Dataset has been gathered for this analysis from the freely accessible UCI machine study repository (Thabtah, 2017) (Thabtah et al., 2017); (Murthy, 2001). Autistic spectrum disorder data for children, dataset and 292 instances and 21 characteristics such as patients' age, gender, nationality were used in this study. The patient had a birth problem with Yaundice, Any family member had widespread developmental disabilities, Who the experiment is done, The property where the customer lives, Screening application previously used by the consumer, Form of screening, Reaction focused on methods of sampling, Multivariate Score.

PROPOSED METHODOLOGY

The proposed work flow diagram that includes pre-processing data, planning and testing using classification techniques with specified models, assessment results and prediction of ASD is presented in Figure 1. The R2020a MATLAB performs this study.

PRE-PROCESSING OF DATA

Data preprocessing (Reyana et al, 2020), (Kaur & Kautish, 2019) is a way of transforming raw data into meaningful and comprehensible formats. Real world statistics are usually inaccurate and incoherent, as they contain many mistakes and zero values. Good pre-processed data also delivers good performance. Incorrect and non-compatible data, i.e., handling lost values, detailing detections, discretification of data, data reduction, etc, are used for different data preprocessing methods. The missing values issues were addressed by an imputation approach in these data sets.

Figure 1. Proposed ASD Identification system

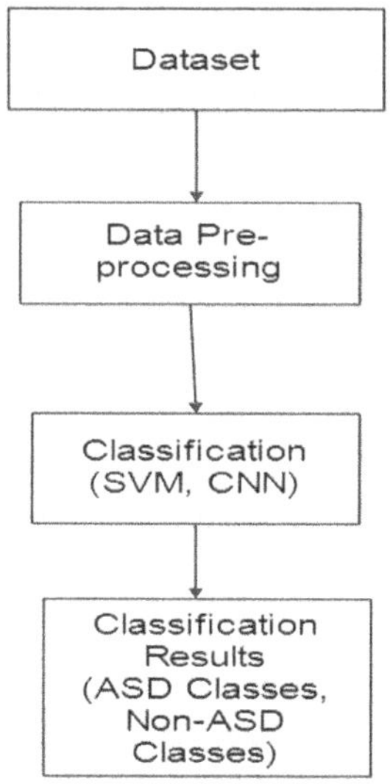

TRAINING AND TESTING SET

The entire dataset was divided into two sections, i.e., 70% and 30%, one section is the data set for preparation, the other part is the data set for research.

SUPPORT VECTOR MACHINE (SVM)

A support vector machine (SVM) is a monitoring machine learning model (Reyana & Kautish, 2021) which uses two group classification issues classifying algorithms. They will categories the new text after providing an SVM model sets of named training data for each type. This does not trigger the overfitting issue. SVM divides the class by specifying the limit of judgement (Wong et. al., 2001). The SVM is a data-classification algorithm for predictive analysis that assigns new data elements to one of the labelled groups. SVM is, in most instances, a binary classifier, supposed to contain two potential target values for the data in question (Ioannidis et. al., 2018).

CONVOLUTIONAL NEURAL NETWORK (CNN)

CNN is one of the profound teaching methods used to construct templates for various problems (Fusaro et. al., 2012). It is a human-brain-inspired neural feed network. A

Figure 2. An SVM classifier

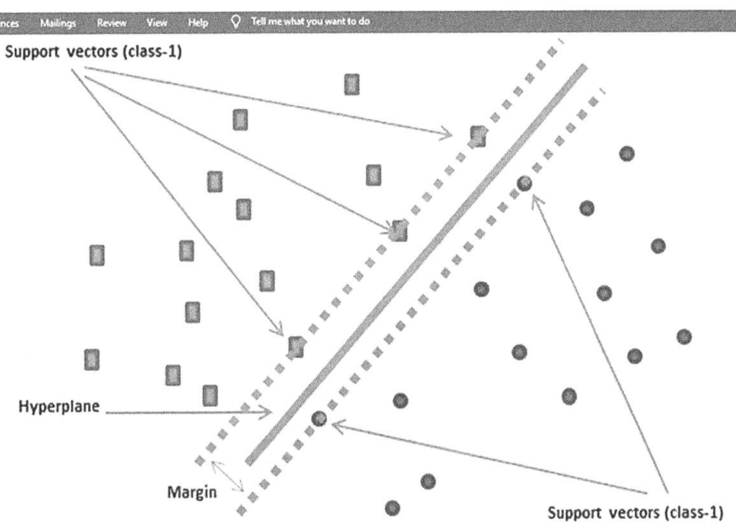

CNN model comprises an input, converting, pooling, one output layer and several other layers - fully linked and standardized. The architecture of CNN has one layer of input. In compute of softmáx active functions, matrix multiplication, followed by the bias offset, can be used. A simple CNN chart is given below:

RESULTS AND DISCUSSION

The results are calculated by the two classification devices SVM and Convolution neural network (CNN) in accuracy, precision, retrieval and f-score. How specific the model is conditioned depends on the outcomes. The proposed methodology is done on the results for children's dataset in autistic spectrum disorder testing. MATLAB Version R2015 was used to perform experiments. Error rating and

Figure 3. Basic structure of a CNN model

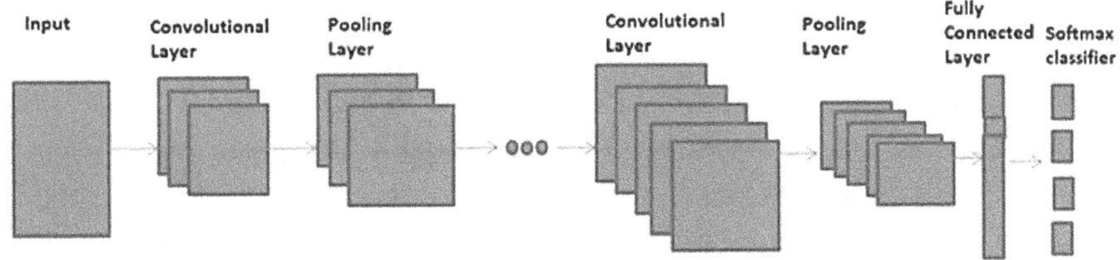

accuracy functions were used to measure efficiency as the metrics. Error rate and precision can be arithmetically determined

Precision= NR_IR / TN_IR (1)

where TN_IR = Total number of images retrieved

NR_IR = Number of relevant images retrieved

The two classifiers supporting vector machine (SVM) and the Convolution Neural Network are the subject of experiments (CNN). The error rate and accuracy in the proposed procedure have been measured and the implications of this classification analysed. The highest success findings for a CNN (Convolution Neural Network) classification were obtained for autism spectrum disorder screening data for infants.

PERFORMANCE METRICS

Output measurement is necessary to decide how a classification model operates successfully to accomplish an objective. The feasibility and efficiency of the study dataset classification model was measured by the performance assessment approaches. The right steps must be chosen to evaluate model performance like accuracy, precision, reminder and f-score. In the following calculations the metrics of performance are used:

Accuracy

Precision determines whether or not the formula you used forecasts better results. It will demonstrate to us automatically whether a model is well trained and how it works. However, in the running program, it does not provide further details about the issue.

Accuracy = (true positives + true negatives)/ (total examples) (2)

Precision

When the good aspects are expected in our present model, accuracy helps confirm it. Precision allows one to assess whether false-positive costs are high. Therefore, if the market dilemma requires the identification of an object, these effects will estimate the same object in the input picture if we have a very low accuracy model.

Precision = (true positives)/ (true positives + false positives) (3)

Recall

Recall allows us to find out if the cost of false negative is high. What if we need to search other items as part of our dilemma. If several images contain different artefacts, results in a single image can be different.

Recall = (true positives)/ (true positives + false negatives) ...... (4)

F-Score

F-score is useful for calculating the accuracy of the test. The precision and the recall are taken into account, so F score is deemed perfect when 1 and absolute loss at 0.

F-score = 2 x (true positives) / (true positives + false negatives) .... (5)

Preliminary results of various machine learning algorithms with all selection functions have been provided for children with ASD screening data. All 21 attributes are chosen to find the exactness, consistency, reminder and file value of the expected model. RBF Kernel with a gamma value of 0.1 was used for SVM. In CNN, softmax activation of 195 epochs is included. The general success metrics of both classifications with data sets are seen in depth in Table 1.

Table 1. Overall results for children's autistic spectrum screening

Classifier	Accuracy (%)	Precision	Recall	F-score
SVM	97.02	0.97	0.1	0.92
CNN	98.94	0.99	0.1	0.96

Evaluation of multiple ASD children's diagnostic machine learning models showed consistency in the initial dataset. The predictive accuracy of CNN and SVM was stated to be 98.94% and 97.02% respectively on the first data collection.

Table 2. ASD data accuracy outcomes for children

Classifiers	Accuracy
Support Vector Machine (SVM)	97.02
Convolutional Neural Network (CNN)	98.94

CONCLUSION

In this paper, two machine learning approaches have been used for the diagnosis of Autism Spectrum Disorder. Diverse criteria have been used for success assessment in nonclinical data set analysis of ASD detection models. This dilemma has a better CNN classification outcome rather than SVM with all its characteristics after treating the missing values. The CNN classifier has reached a high degree of precision compared with the SVM technique. These results clearly show that an autism-spektrum condition CNN model should be used instead of a conventional machine learning classification, as was suggested in previous research.

REFERENCES

Bone, D., Goodwin, M. S., Black, M. P., Lee, C. C., Audhkhasi, K., & Narayanan, S. (2015). Applying machine learning to facilitate autism diagnostics: Pitfalls and promises. *Journal of Autism and Developmental Disorders, 45*(5), 1121–1136. doi:10.100710803-014-2268-6 PMID:25294649

Bone, D., Lee, C. C., Black, M. P., Williams, M. E., Lee, S., Levitt, P., & Narayanan, S. (2014). The psychologist as an interlocutor in autism spectrum disorder assessment: Insights from a study of spontaneous prosody. *Journal of Speech, Language, and Hearing Research: JSLHR, 57*(4), 1162–1177. doi:10.1044/2014_JSLHR-S-13-0062 PMID:24686340

Constantino, J. N., Lavesser, P. D., Zhang, Y. I., Abbacchi, A. M., Gray, T., & Todd, R. D. (2007). Rapid quantitative assessment of autistic social impairment by classroom teachers. *Journal of the American Academy of Child and Adolescent Psychiatry, 46*(12), 1668–1676. doi:10.1097/chi.0b013e318157cb23 PMID:18030089

John, G. H., & Langley, P. (2013). *Estimating continuous distributions in Bayesian classifiers.* arXiv preprint arXiv:1302.4964.

Kaur, R., & Kautish, S. (2019). Multimodal sentiment analysis: A survey and comparison. *International Journal of Service Science, Management, Engineering, and Technology, 10*(2), 38–58. doi:10.4018/IJSSMET.2019040103

Keerthi, S. S., Shevade, S. K., Bhattacharyya, C., & Murthy, K. R. K. (2001). Improvements to Platt's SMO algorithm for SVM classifier design. *Neural Computation, 13*(3), 637–649. doi:10.1162/089976601300014493

Kosmicki, J. A., Sochat, V., Duda, M., & Wall, D. P. (2015). Searching for a minimal set of behaviors for autism detection through feature selection-based machine learning. *Translational Psychiatry, 5*(2), e514–e514. doi:10.1038/tp.2015.7 PMID:25710120

Li, B., Sharma, A., Meng, J., Purushwalkam, S., & Gowen, E. (2017). Applying machine learning to identify autistic adults using imitation: An exploratory study. *PLoS One, 12*(8), e0182652. doi:10.1371/journal.pone.0182652 PMID:28813454

Liu, B., Ma, Y., & Wong, C. K. (2001). Classification using association rules: weaknesses and enhancements. In *Data mining for scientific and engineering applications* (pp. 591–605). Springer. doi:10.1007/978-1-4615-1733-7_30

Mythili, M. S., & Shanavas, A. M. (2014). A study on Autism spectrum disorders using classification techniques. *International Journal of Soft Computing and Engineering, 4*(5), 88–91.

Ozdenizci, O., Cumpanasoiu, C., Mazefsky, C., Siegel, M., Erdogmus, D., & Ioannidis, S. (2018). *Time-series prediction of proximal aggression on set in minimally-verbal youth with autism spectrum disorder using physiological biosignals.* arXiv:1809.09948.

Pace, G. M., Iwata, B. A., Edwards, G. L., & McCosh, K. C. (1986). Stimulus fading and transfer in the treatment of self-restraint and self-injurious behavior. *Journal of Applied Behavior Analysis, 19*(4), 381–389. doi:10.1901/jaba.1986.19-381 PMID:3804871

Pelios, L., Morren, J., Tesch, D., & Axelrod, S. (1999). The impact of functional analysis methodology on treatment choice for self-injurious and aggressive behavior. *Journal of Applied Behavior Analysis, 32*(2), 185–195. doi:10.1901/jaba.1999.32-185 PMID:10396771

Plötz, T., Hammerla, N. Y., & Olivier, P. (2011). Feature learning for activity recognition in ubiquitous computing. *IJCAI Proceedings-International Joint Conference on Artificial Intelligence.*

Plötz, T., Hammerla, N. Y., Rozga, A., Reavis, A., Call, N., & Abowd, G. D. (2012). Automatic assessment of problem behavior in individuals with developmental disabilities. *Proceedings of the 2012 ACM conference on ubiquitous computing*. 10.1145/2370216.2370276

Poliker, R. (2006). Pattern recognition. In *Wiley Encyclopaedia of biomedical engineering*. Wiley. doi:10.1002/9780471740360.ebs0904

Preece, S. J., Goulermas, J. Y., Kenney, L. P., Howard, D., Meijer, K., & Crompton, R. (2009). Activityidentificationusingbody-mountedsensors—A review of classification techniques. *Physiological Measurement*, *30*(4), R1–R33. doi:10.1088/0967-3334/30/4/R01 PMID:19342767

Pugliese, C. E., Kenworthy, L., Bal, V. H., Wallace, G. L., Yerys, B.E., & Maddox, B. B. (2015). Replication and comparison ofthe newly proposed ADOS-2, module 4 algorithm in ASD with-out ID: A multi-site study. *Journal of Autism and Developmental Disorders, 45*(12), 3919–3931. . doi:10.100710803-015-2586-3

Rad, N. M., Furlanello, C., & Kessler, F. B. (2016). Applying deep learning to stereo typical motor movement detection in autism spectrum disorders. *2016 IEEE 16th international conference on data mining workshops*.

Rani, S., & Kautish, S. (2018, June). Association clustering and time series based data mining in continuous data for diabetes prediction. In *2018 second international conference on intelligent computing and control systems (ICICCS)* (pp. 1209-1214). IEEE. 10.1109/ICCONS.2018.8662909

Rani, S., & Kautish, S. (2018). Application of data mining techniques for prediction of diabetes-A review. International Journal of Scientific Research in Computer Science. *Engineering and Information Technology*, *3*(3), 1996–2004.

Reyana, A., & Kautish, S. (2021). *Corona virus-related Disease Pandemic: A Review on Machine Learning Approaches and Treatment Trials on Diagnosed Population for Future Clinical Decision Support*. Current Medical Imaging.

Reyana, A., Krishnaprasath, V. T., Kautish, S., Panigrahi, R., & Shaik, M. (2020). Decision-making on the existence of soft exudates in diabetic retinopathy. *International Journal of Computer Applications in Technology*, *64*(4), 375–381. doi:10.1504/IJCAT.2020.112684

Saini, G. K., Chouhan, H., Kori, S., Gupta, A., Shabaz, M., Jagota, V., & Singh, B. K. (2021). Recognition of Human Sentiment from Image using Machine Learning. *Annals of the Romanian Society for Cell Biology*, *25*(5), 1802–1808.

Sampathkumar, A., Rastogi, R., Arukonda, S., Shankar, A., Kautish, S., & Sivaram, M. (2020). An efficient hybrid methodology for detection of cancer-causing gene using CSC for micro array data. *Journal of Ambient Intelligence and Humanized Computing*, *11*(11), 4743–4751. doi:10.100712652-020-01731-7

Singh, P., & Dhiman, G. (2017, December). A fuzzy-LP approach in time series forecasting. In *International Conference on Pattern Recognition and Machine Intelligence* (pp. 243-253). Springer. 10.1007/978-3-319-69900-4_31

Singh, P., & Dhiman, G. (2018). A hybrid fuzzy time series forecasting model based on granular computing and bio-inspired optimization approaches. *Journal of Computational Science*, *27*, 370–385. doi:10.1016/j.jocs.2018.05.008

Singh, P., & Dhiman, G. (2018). Uncertainty representation using fuzzy-entropy approach: Special application in remotely sensed high-resolution satellite images (RSHRSIs). *Applied Soft Computing*, *72*, 121–139. doi:10.1016/j.asoc.2018.07.038

Thabtah, F. (2017). *ASDTests. A mobile app for ASD screening*. Academic Press.

Thabtah, F. (2017). Autism spectrum disorder screening: Machine learning adaptation and DSM-5 fulfillment. *Proceedings of the 1st International Conference on Medical and Health Informatics (MDPI)*, 1–6.

Thabtah, F. (2019). Machine learning in autistic spectrum disorder behavioral research: A review and ways forward. *Informatics for Health & Social Care*, *44*(3), 278–297. doi:10.1080/17538157.2017.1399132 PMID:29436887

Thabtah, F., Kamalov, F., & Rajab, K. (2018). A new computational intelligence approach to detect autistic features for autism screening. *International Journal of Medical Informatics*, *117*, 112–124. doi:10.1016/j.ijmedinf.2018.06.009 PMID:30032959

Thabtah, F. F. (2017). *Autistic spectrum disorder screening data for children data set*. Academic Press.

Vaishali, R., & Sasikala, R. (2018). A machine learning based approach to classify autism with optimum behaviour sets. *Int. J. Eng. Technol*, *7*, 18.

Wall, D. P., Dally, R., Luyster, R., Jung, J. Y., & DeLuca, T. F. (2012). Use of artificial intelligence to shorten the behavioral diagnosis of autism. *PLoS One*, *7*(8), e43855. doi:10.1371/journal.pone.0043855 PMID:22952789

Wall, D. P., Kosmicki, J., Deluca, T. F., Harstad, E., & Fusaro, V. A. (2012). Use of machine learning to shorten observation-based screening and diagnosis of autism. *Translational Psychiatry*, *2*(4), e100–e100. doi:10.1038/tp.2012.10 PMID:22832900

Chapter 6 ML-PASD: Predict Autism Spectrum Disorder by Machine Learning Approach

Vishal Jagota
Madanapalle Institute of Technology and Science, India

Vinay Bhatia
Chandigarh Engineering College, India

Luis Vives
https://orcid.org/0000-0003-0280-2990
Universidad Peruana de Ciencias Aplicadas, Lima, Peru

Arun B. Prasad
https://orcid.org/0000-0002-6108-9219
Nirma University, Ahmedabad, India

ABSTRACT

Autism spectrum disorder (ASD) is growing faster than ever before. Autism detection is costly and time intensive with screening procedures. Autism can be detected at an early stage by the development of artificial intelligence and machine learning (ML). While a number of experiments using many approaches were conducted, these studies provided no conclusion as to the prediction of autism characteristics in various age groups. This chapter is therefore intended to suggest an accurate MLASD predictive model based on the ML methodology to prevent ASD for people of all ages. It is a method for prediction. This survey was conducted to develop and assess ASD prediction in an artificial neural network (ANN). AQ-10 data collection was used to test the proposed pattern. The findings of the evaluation reveal that the proposed prediction model has improved results in terms of consistency, specificity, sensitivity, and dataset accuracy.

DOI: 10.4018/978-1-7998-7460-7.ch006

INTRODUCTION

Diagnoses of ASD based on behavioural characteristics (Omar et al., 2019), although in many but most cases, the exact cause of ASD is not understood (Cruz & Wishart, 2006). Reliable determination of ASD is a big problem for ASD monitoring schemes and broad studies of ASD generally.

Although stringent ASD diagnostic instruments do exist, clinicians use a range of daily practical resources and approaches (Khan et al., 2017). It is also impossible to identify ASD using "gold-standard" clinic-based practises for large-scale or population-based trials. Many trials in epidemiology are based somewhat, and often only, on current "administrative" ASD grading designations: ICD 9, billing codes, special education or the autism related disorder insurance eligibility (e.g., Medicaid) (Wall et al., 2012; Bone et al., 2016). There is a substantial inconsistency in the use of these classifications in the United States. These programmes are not universal in determining all persons that follow the population ASD requirements and their main goals are ensuring adequate provision of care to people rather than classifying disabilities (Allison et al., 2012; Thabtah, 2017).

The data used to test atypical variances in children with and without ASD in face expressions (Hauck and Kliewer, 2017). Using knowledge theory, mathematical analysis and time series simulation, six facial responses were securitised. Researchers have recently embraced data analytics as a diagnostic method for ASD in refinement and implementation. The possibility of grouping in the different domains has been revealed by being an effective computer tool (Bekerom, 2017). Therefore, some literature has used machine learning techniques in order to distinguish persons with and without ASD that are discriminating against neurons (Wall, 2012), behaviour indicators (Heinsfeld et al., 2018) and (Saini et al., 2021) sentiments respectively. The effect of the eyes on children with high- or low-risk children at high-ASD levels. Computing approaches were applied, such as 0.61 accurate discrimination analysis for the discriminating functions, 0.64 precision support for vector machine, and a 0.56 accuracy linear discrimination analysis. The Autism-diagnostic interview and the social responsiveness level were revised, SMV machine learning categories were extended to a leading sample of people with or without ASD, and positive findings were obtained (Bone et al., 2015).

(Kosmicki et al., 2015) used artificial neural networks to create a predictive model based on a data collection of 22 possible risk elements for pregnancy in the development of autism (Omar et al., 2019). The predictive accuracy of the artificial neural network was 83 percent. Their research promoted the use of ANNs as an outstanding diagnosis monitoring method for ASD, and welcomed them. The highest level of accuracy achieved to date is 95.07 percent for SVM (Reyana et al, 2020).

Autism diagnosis takes a great deal of time and expenses. Earlier diagnosis of autism behaviours, such as verbal, nonverbal speech, perseverance, physical skills, repeated behaviour, sensory treatment and social awareness etc. may be helpful when administering early medicine to patients, as seen in Figure 1. It may help prevent further deterioration of the health of the patient, and reduce the long-term costs of late diagnosis. Autism characteristics in a person and whether or not an extensive autism evaluation is needed.

This research aims to formulate a model of autism prediction using ML techniques and create a smartphone app that can accurately predict the autism traits of a person of any generation. This thesis focuses on the development of an autism screening application to predict ASD characteristics of individuals between the ages of 4-11 years, 12-17 years and 18 years and older.

The key problem with a perfect SMM recognition is the identification of the most significant characteristics which carry stereotypical behaviour by means of an automated feature extraction technique from accelerometers. Another problem is personalization caused by variability within and between subjects (Liaw and Wiener, 2002). Intrasubject variances can in fact be explained by variations in severity, length and frequency of SMM in any atypical subject (subject of the automotive spectrums) whereas variances between SMMs among different atypical subjects can be explained by inter-subject variances (Bone, 2015).

An adaptive method (Sampathkumar et al, 2020) is thus essential in order to generalise all SMMs through individuals and to respond to new SMM behaviour. These problems can be solved with profound SMM identification learning strategies.

Figure 1. Symptoms of ASD

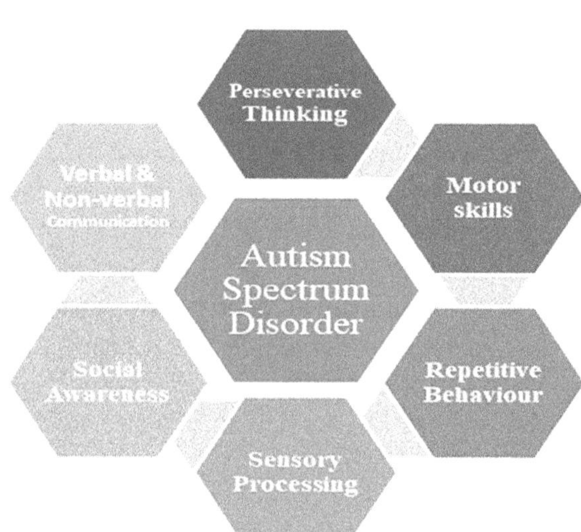

We train two CNN models inside the subjects in times and frequency areas whose parameters are selected on the basis of the properties of the SMM input.

We create a global, fast and lightweight SMM Detection Platform that combines an SVM classifier with an information transferral platform that delivers promising results by adjusting SMMs of some unusual new topic. One benefit of the platform is the use of only few labelled data on this atypical topic as well as large numbers of other atypical topics, thus solving a "actual-life" medical problem linked to the lack of supervised SMMs by applying cross-domain transmission training (e.g., from a field other than the target domain for the SMM).

Machine learning is an IT field, and in particular an artificial intelligence branch. Its key feature is its ability to learn from previous inputs and to refine new outputs. We can process a huge amount of information using machine learning techniques (Wall et al., 2012). In a recent report, Stevens et al. defined subgroups of ASD with Linear Analysis Machine Learning Processes (LDA) about the kinetic nature of walking with predictions of 78.05% accuracy and a low error level (Wall et al., 2012).

A machine-learning approach (Reyana & Kautish, 2021) has recently been applied to differentiate ASD persons from non-ASD people and has shown considerable promise. Mechanical learning in computer science as a branch of artificial intelligence is a process that trains a computer algorithm to analyse a number of observations and statistically acquire latent patterns without being specifically programmed. It is applied to brain function (Vahia, 2013) and ET (Liu et al., 2016) and it has been applied to behaviour (Butler et al., 2015).

As we have said, the available diagnostic methods (Rani & Kautish, 2018) therefore require several hours of waiting and test a small percentage of cases (Thabtah, 2017). Moreover, given the symptoms are time-changed and re-evaluated, the entire thing can be monotonous and stressful for the children and their parents. Furthermore, the scales are not fully quantitative, meaning that the conclusions may be wrong (Bone et al., 2014). The use of artificial intelligence, a new approach to increase accuracy and efficiency during diagnosis of autism, will improve this pressure.

An AMN (Kaur & Kautish, 2019) is built on an artificial neuron series of linked units or nodes that roughly model the neurons in the biological brain. Each connection can send a signal to other neurons, like the synapses in a biological brain. An artificial neuron, which absorbs a signal, will then process it and signal connected neurons. The "signal" at a link is a real number, and each neuron's output is calculated with a certain non-linear function of its inputs' amount. The links are known as the sides. Usually, neurons and edges weigh down to the progress of learning. The weight increases the signal power at a link or reduces it. Intelligence in artificial form is connected to the development of computer systems that imitate human behaviour but still have the capacity to learn, adapt, consider and resolve environmental problems. According to the inventor of the word "artificial intelligence," John McCarthy, the technology involved in creating smart machines is AI. An outstanding concept is "the analysis of ideas that make machines intelligent" (Thabtah et al., 2017). Artificial intelligence is not limited to simply performing commands but can carry out difficult tasks automatically, which require time and effort for human beings (Li et al., 2017).

LITERATURE REVIEW

(Mythili and Shanavas, 2014) Tried cancer with ML to predict whether or not an individual is diabetic. Alternative Tree of Decision (ADTree) to reduce screen time and to quickly diagnose ASD traits. They used Autism Diagnostic Interview, revised procedure (ADI-R), and obtained high precision with data of 790 people. However, the evaluation was restricted within 5-17 years and ASD for various age groups was not predicted (children, adolescent and adults).

Prediction mechanisms have been investigated by a study of children with autism after 3 years of clinical observation and therapies and behavioral treatment (Kosmicki et al., 2015). Machine learning models were used to research psychiatric, developmental, social and demographic components that influence the prognosis of autism children. They sought to forecast short-term autism outcomes and to identify clinical and personal causes affecting symptomatic progress. In the beginning, data from control lists such as Autistic Behavior Checklist and Aberrant Checklist were gathered and evaluated using the Naïve Bayes, Generalized Linear Model, Logistic Regression and Decision Tree algorithms. They then correlated the positive or bad effects with the frequency of the therapeutic variables. To explain the data, they decided to use a decision book. This approach will allow clinicians to distinguish sub-classes in autism cases, as well as other complex neurodevelopment conditions even though the research findings are preliminary. Decision trees are trees used for classification of occurrences. Each tree node represents one instant characteristic and every branch represents the result. The connection paths are the rules of classification. It is a reality that information can be visualized using decision-making trees.

(Thabtah, 2017) Applying 91.02 per cent sensitivity and 62 per cent speciality ML for the same reason and using a support vector machine (SVM). They used 1072 ASD persons and 780 NON-ASD persons for their study. Because of its wide age range (from four to 55 years) its study was not approved as a screening method for all age groups used as a 'Red Flag' screening technique for autism spectrum quoting ASDs for children and adults.

(John and Langley,2013) A deep learning algorithm and a neural network were employed to classify ASD patients using the Autism Imaging Data Exchange's broad brain imaging data collection and to achieve a mean accuracy range of between 67%

and 82%. Average accuracy of the SVM classifier was 67% while the mean accuracy of the Random Forest classifier was 89%.

It is clear from the literature review that, while a variety of studies in this area has been performed, the researchers have not concluded decisively using the ML method to generalize autism diagnostic testing in terms of age ranges. Different methods and procedures for autism screening test were already adapted but none for different age ranges were modified in the form of app-based approach.

Proposed MLASD Method

The aim of the studies using machine learning was to facilitate and time consuming the evaluation process of ASD. However, it is vital to take the conceptual and analytical details into account when implementing these approaches. For e.g., where the psychometric device is not fully managed it is necessary to consider the consequences of the validity. Interdisciplinary approaches are currently still needed. Consequently, informatics specialists who develop algorithms should be able to understand novel technology, as well as autism. In ASD study the cooperation of many areas seems fruitful.

By using ANN machine-learning methods focused on knowledge gathered from prospective ASD patients' medical forms. The detection system consisted of hand-written, semi-structured and unstructured medical forms that later were translated into digital formats. Expert physicians assess the test outcomes. Furthermore, another new AI application, using the ability to measure stereotype behavior in autism children with modern smart watches. It used an adaptive accelerometer to track individuals with an autistic spectrum's normal conduct.AI Hardware includes an intelligent watch and a mobile phone, which captures the accelerometer's sensory data as well

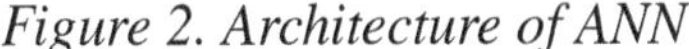
Figure 2. Architecture of ANN

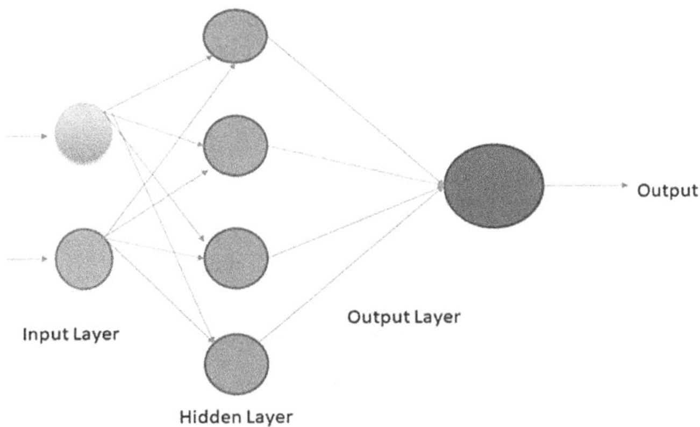

as machine learning algorithms, which track and identify repeating competencies. This technology will also allow doctors to decide for themselves. Data is used for the identification of autistic conducts as the result and the judgement.

The information provided on the ANN model is the user information displayed as a 1D tensor with twelve coefficients, including user responses to ten behavioral issues, participant age, sex, whether the user is jaundiced and any family ASD history. We combined datasets from various age publications and assembled one dataset that represents the complete data from the various categories of age. Initial data for the training of ANN were primarily derived from the AQ-10 dataset. As one of the separate variables considered during ANN instruction, the age of the pupil learns to better link age with the class of ASD when seeking ASD characteristics, among other variables. The data will be pre-processed with one-hot encoding and dummy variables removed and user age presentation in size 3 bins. The data pre-treatment process increases the dimension of the input tensor from 12 to 34 coefficients. This data is subsequently feed to the ANN model for results.

RESULTS AND DISCUSSIONS

Dataset AQ-10 was used for the accuracy evaluation of the proposed predictive model. The predictor model created could be used to recommend potential autism traits to people who are not diagnosed. The model suggests a human in Table 1 with two potential parameters:

The methodology applied has been tested with three age groups (child, teen, and adult) and the findings have been compared on the basis of the criteria described above. AQ-10 dataset consists of three separate datasets based on concerns about the AQ-10 screening method. The three datasets include data from 4-11 years of age (child), 12-16 years of age (adults) and 18 or over (adults) of age as seen in Table 2. To determine when a person needs referral to be made to a full autism evaluation, use AQ-10 or autism spectrum quotient method.

Screening AQ-10 dataset-based questions are focused on various fields, such as attention to detail, care change, conversation, creativity and social engagement. The

Table 1. Possible parameters of user categories

Parameter	Yes/No
User has possible autism traits and requires comprehensive autism assessment	Yes
User does not have autism traits	No

Table 2. Dataset instances

Age Group	Outcome
Child (4-11) years	292
Adolescent (12-16) years	104
Adult (18 or above) years	704

Table 3. Accuracy obtained on AQ-10 dataset

Age Group	Accuracy (%)
Child	96.06
Adolescent	97.78
Adult	93.54

question score system is that for each of 10 questions only one point can be scored. On each question, users can score by 0 or 1 point, depending on their response and by using the AQ-10 data set they can score 96,06 percent, 97,78 percent and 93,54 percent for boy, teen and adult persons.

For computing the output parameters for the applied methodology, AQ-10 datasets were used. All other data except the instance will be used as training data when forecasting an instance. The findings indicates that, for each output parameter; for

Figure 3. Accuracy obtained

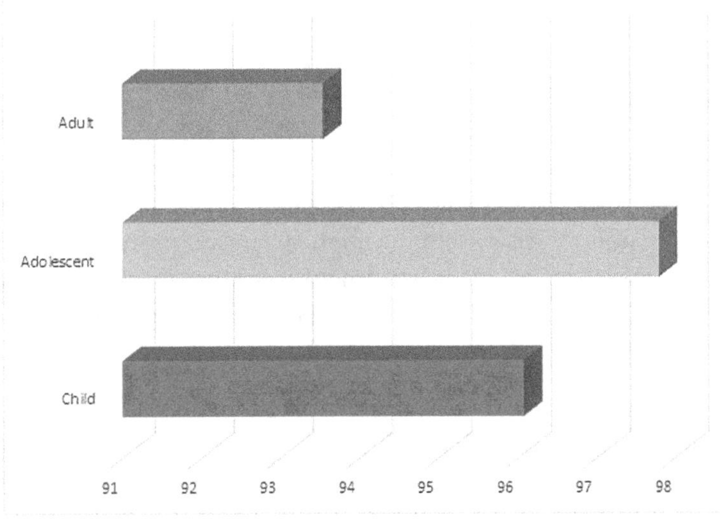

each group of participants, the MLASD prediction model proposed produces better results in comparison with the two existing versions. The proposed prediction model again demonstrated better outcomes to adults and adolescents, while AQ-10 data sets were used to train prediction models for children, young people and adults. The AQ-10 dataset forecast results are shown in Figure 3. Compared to state-of-the-art datasets, the precision of the AQ-10 is higher.

CONCLUSION

Autism with 96.06%, 97.78%, and 93.54% for children, teenagers and adults, can be predicted by the proposed model, by using the AQ-10 dataset. This was a higher success than the other current autism screening technique. In addition, the proposed model will predict autism characteristics for various age groups The results of these studies provide the autism traits of various ages with an efficient and accurate solution. Since autism is quite an expensive and long procedure, the diagnosis is often postponed because children and teenagers have trouble identifying autism. By means of autism checks a person should be directed early on, so that the situation does not worsen and the costs of delayed diagnosis are lowered.

REFERENCES

Allison, C., Auyeung, B., & Baron-Cohen, S. (2012). Toward brief "red flags" for autism screening: The short autism spectrum quotient and the short quantitative checklist in 1,000 cases and 3,000 controls. *Journal of the American Academy of Child and Adolescent Psychiatry*, *51*(2), 202–212. doi:10.1016/j.jaac.2011.11.003 PMID:22265366

Bekerom, B. (2017). Using machine learning for detection of autism spectrum disorder. In *Proc. 20th Student Conf. IT* (pp. 1-7). Academic Press.

Bone, D., Bishop, S. L., Black, M. P., Goodwin, M. S., Lord, C., & Narayanan, S. S. (2016). Use of machine learning to improve autism screening and diagnostic instruments: Effectiveness, efficiency, and multi-instrument fusion. *Journal of Child Psychology and Psychiatry, and Allied Disciplines*, *57*(8), 927–937. doi:10.1111/jcpp.12559 PMID:27090613

Bone, D., Goodwin, M. S., Black, M. P., Lee, C. C., Audhkhasi, K., & Narayanan, S. (2015). Applying machine learning to facilitate autism diagnostics: Pitfalls and promises. *Journal of Autism and Developmental Disorders*, *45*(5), 1121–1136. doi:10.100710803-014-2268-6 PMID:25294649

Bone, D., Lee, C. C., Black, M. P., Williams, M. E., Lee, S., Levitt, P., & Narayanan, S. (2014). The psychologist as an interlocutor in autism spectrum disorder assessment: Insights from a study of spontaneous prosody. *Journal of Speech, Language, and Hearing Research: JSLHR*, *57*(4), 1162–1177. doi:10.1044/2014_JSLHR-S-13-0062 PMID:24686340

Butler, M. G., Rafi, S. K., Hossain, W., Stephan, D. A., & Manzardo, A. M. (2015). Whole exome sequencing in females with autism implicates novel and candidate genes. *International Journal of Molecular Sciences*, *16*(1), 1312–1335. doi:10.3390/ijms16011312 PMID:25574603

Cruz, J. A., & Wishart, D. S. (2006). Applications of machine learning in cancer prediction and prognosis. *Cancer Informatics*, *2*. doi:10.1177/117693510600200030 PMID:19458758

Hauck, F., & Kliewer, N. (2017). Machine Learning for Autism Diagnostics: Applying Support Vector Classification. *Int'l Conf. Health Informatics and Medical Systems.*

Heinsfeld, A. S., Franco, A. R., Craddock, R. C., Buchweitz, A., & Meneguzzi, F. (2018). Identification of autism spectrum disorder using deep learning and the ABIDE dataset. *NeuroImage. Clinical*, *17*, 16–23. doi:10.1016/j.nicl.2017.08.017 PMID:29034163

John, G. H., & Langley, P. (2013). *Estimating continuous distributions in Bayesian classifiers*. arXiv preprint arXiv:1302.4964.

Kaur, R., & Kautish, S. (2019). Multimodal sentiment analysis: A survey and comparison. *International Journal of Service Science, Management, Engineering, and Technology*, *10*(2), 38–58. doi:10.4018/IJSSMET.2019040103

Khan, N. S., Muaz, M. H., Kabir, A., & Islam, M. N. (2017, December). Diabetes predicting mhealth application using machine learning. In *2017 IEEE International WIE Conference on Electrical and Computer Engineering (WIECON-ECE)* (pp. 237-240). IEEE. 10.1109/WIECON-ECE.2017.8468885

Kosmicki, J. A., Sochat, V., Duda, M., & Wall, D. P. (2015). Searching for a minimal set of behaviors for autism detection through feature selection-based machine learning. *Translational Psychiatry*, *5*(2), e514–e514. doi:10.1038/tp.2015.7 PMID:25710120

Li, B., Sharma, A., Meng, J., Purushwalkam, S., & Gowen, E. (2017). Applying machine learning to identify autistic adults using imitation: An exploratory study. *PLoS One*, *12*(8), e0182652. doi:10.1371/journal.pone.0182652 PMID:28813454

Liaw, A., & Wiener, M. (2002). Classification and regression by random Forest. *R News*, *2*(3), 18–22.

Liu, W., Li, M., & Yi, L. (2016). Identifying children with autism spectrum disorder based on their face processing abnormality: A machine learning framework. *Autism Research*, *9*(8), 888–898. doi:10.1002/aur.1615 PMID:27037971

Mythili, M. S., & Shanavas, A. M. (2014). A study on Autism spectrum disorders using classification techniques. *International Journal of Soft Computing and Engineering*, *4*(5), 88–91.

Omar, K. S., Mondal, P., Khan, N. S., Rizvi, M. R. K., & Islam, M. N. (2019). A machine learning approach to predict autism spectrum disorder. In *2019 International Conference on Electrical, Computer and Communication Engineering (ECCE)* (pp. 1-6). IEEE. 10.1109/ECACE.2019.8679454

Rani, S., & Kautish, S. (2018). Association clustering and time series based data mining in continuous data for diabetes prediction. In *2018 second international conference on intelligent computing and control systems (ICICCS)* (pp. 1209-1214). IEEE. 10.1109/ICCONS.2018.8662909

Rani, S., & Kautish, S. (2018). Application of data mining techniques for prediction of diabetes-A review. International Journal of Scientific Research in Computer Science. *Engineering and Information Technology*, *3*(3), 1996–2004.

Reyana, A., & Kautish, S. (2021). *Corona virus-related Disease Pandemic: A Review on Machine Learning Approaches and Treatment Trials on Diagnosed Population for Future Clinical Decision Support*. Current Medical Imaging.

Reyana, A., Krishnaprasath, V. T., Kautish, S., Panigrahi, R., & Shaik, M. (2020). Decision-making on the existence of soft exudates in diabetic retinopathy. *International Journal of Computer Applications in Technology*, *64*(4), 375–381. doi:10.1504/IJCAT.2020.112684

Saini, G. K., Chouhan, H., Kori, S., Gupta, A., Shabaz, M., Jagota, V., & Singh, B. K. (2021). Recognition of Human Sentiment from Image using Machine Learning. *Annals of the Romanian Society for Cell Biology*, *25*(5), 1802–1808.

Sampathkumar, A., Rastogi, R., Arukonda, S., Shankar, A., Kautish, S., & Sivaram, M. (2020). An efficient hybrid methodology for detection of cancer-causing gene using CSC for micro array data. *Journal of Ambient Intelligence and Humanized Computing*, *11*(11), 4743–4751.

Singh, P., & Dhiman, G. (2017, December). A fuzzy-LP approach in time series forecasting. In *International Conference on Pattern Recognition and Machine Intelligence* (pp. 243-253). Springer. 10.1007/978-3-319-69900-4_31

Singh, P., & Dhiman, G. (2018). A hybrid fuzzy time series forecasting model based on granular computing and bio-inspired optimization approaches. *Journal of Computational Science*, *27*, 370–385. doi:10.1016/j.jocs.2018.05.008

Singh, P., & Dhiman, G. (2018). Uncertainty representation using fuzzy-entropy approach: Special application in remotely sensed high-resolution satellite images (RSHRSIs). *Applied Soft Computing*, *72*, 121–139. doi:10.1016/j.asoc.2018.07.038

Thabtah, F. (2017, May). Autism spectrum disorder screening: Machine learning adaptation and DSM-5 fulfillment. *Proceedings of the 1st International Conference on Medical and Health Informatics (MDPI)*, 1–6.

Vahia, V. N. (2013). Diagnostic and statistical manual of mental disorders 5: A quick glance. *Indian Journal of Psychiatry*, *55*(3), 220–223. doi:10.4103/0019-5545.117131 PMID:24082241

Wall, D. P., Dally, R., Luyster, R., Jung, J. Y., & DeLuca, T. F. (2012). Use of artificial intelligence to shorten the behavioral diagnosis of autism. *PLoS One*, *7*(8), e43855. doi:10.1371/journal.pone.0043855 PMID:22952789

Wall, D. P., Kosmicki, J., Deluca, T. F., Harstad, E., & Fusaro, V. A. (2012). Use of machine learning to shorten observation-based screening and diagnosis of autism. *Translational Psychiatry*, *2*(4), e100–e100. doi:10.1038/tp.2012.10 PMID:22832900

Chapter 7
Existing Assistive Techniques for Dyslexics: A Systematic Review

Kulwinder Singh
Punjabi University, Baba Jogipeer Neighbourhood, India

Vishal Goyal
Punjabi University, Patiala, India

Parshant Rana
Thapar Institute of Engineering and Technology, India

ABSTRACT

Reading is an essential skill for literacy development in children. But it is a challenge for children with dyslexia because of phonological-core deficits. Poor reading skills have an impact on vocabulary development and to exposure to relevant background knowledge. It affects the ability to interpret what one sees and hears or the ability to link information from different parts of the brain. Dyslexic children face many challenges in their educational life due to reading difficulty. Support to dyslexic children include computer-based applications and multi-sensory methods like text-to-speech and character animation techniques. Some applications provide immediate reading intervention facility. Automatic speech recognition (ASR) is a new platform with immediate intervention for assisting dyslexic children to improve their reading ability. Findings contribute to develop a suitable approach to correct the reading mistakes of dyslexic children. Speech recognition technology provides the most interactive environment between human and machine.

DOI: 10.4018/978-1-7998-7460-7.ch007

INTRODUCTION

Dyslexia is a language based learning disability that affects reading. Dyslexia is most common reading difficulty, it is estimated that one out of 10 children is dyslexic. According International Dyslexia Association 15 to 20% world population detected symptom of dyslexia. Dyslexia has created a problem in processing word-sounds, identify the sound of letters. They have problem in understanding reversal letters and confusion between letters. Result of dyslexia phonics problems in language; reduce reading capability, vocabulary growth, and other knowledge. Table 1 represents some assistive software for dyslexic children to enhance learning ability. Dyslexia may impede child's developing and learning capability. The performance of a dyslexic child is very low: trouble in reading at a good pace without mistake.

Due to difficulty in dyslexic children mastering in reading is a challenge. Very limited research for dyslexic children has been till now in regional languages. We find that dyslexia still not widely known in India and the research on this topic is extremely scarce.

To facilitate learning experience for dyslexics children help is essential needed (Husni & Jamaludin, 2009). People with dyslexia fail to comprehend the text as presented. A dyslexic person does not understand what is written, gives miss-meaning of the passage, and forget the sequence of events (Rahman, et al. 2012). Dyslexia can be managed or sustained with the help of special methods or techniques. Developing computer technologies helps to parents and teachers of dyslexic children in their teaching with easy and efficient manner. Dyslexia mostly affects on school age population around 6% to 17%. FunLexia is an educational game to help dyslexia children to learn Arabic. A heuristic evaluation and speech therapists indicates that FunLexia is supportive tool and promote leaning for children with dyslexia (Ouherrou et al. 2018). Graphogame is a game help to children to read in their local language.

Speech recognition is providing confidence and timing a child to track during read- aloud. The speech recognizer must follow behaviors of students quickly and accurately, when students reading fluently the cursor appear at right time and at right place and pauses when students hesitate. The students receive feedback about their pronunciation (Hagen et al., 2004). Multimedia elements (Sampathkumar et al 2020) are used as guidelines for learning skills in dyslexic students through special instructions.

Assist to dyslexic learners in learning within normal peer group needs an adaptive reading assistance system that is easy to understand. Adaptive reading assistance (Reyana, & Kautish, 2021) allows dyslexic students to reading text documents arbitrary using augmented way such as emphasis on characters, text highlighting, segmenting words. AGENT-DYSL system is adaptive to presentation of individual student and suggest individual for further training (Schmidt & Schneider, 2007).

Watch Me! a reading software designed for young children provide reading practice, sense of reading and comprehension awareness. Speech recognition used to assess students reading ability and gives individual feedback (Williams et al., 2013). ASR providing a reading tutor towards advancing that listen what is read by dyslexic children and give correct or incorrect reading feedback. Dyslexic children read aloud 114 words in Bahasa Melayu and speech recorded. ASR trained based on resulting utterances that transcribed and the pronunciations are modeled (Husni & Jamaluddin, 2008).

Recurrent neural network (Rani, & Kautish, 2018) used for creating speech recognition in Bengali language to find character probabilities. There has been widespread use of speech recognition at beginning of twenty-first century. It is very helpful for persons who have typing difficulty and those with spelling difficulties. Two models for Bengali speech recognition system, first model for recognize spoken language using Convolutional Neural Network (CNN) and second model use recurrent neural network. HMM phoneme and word based models used for training isolated and continuous word speech recognition. The CNN model accuracy convert speech to text is 86.058% and 30000 Bengali words used to train RNN model which converts speech signal into text transcriptions (Islam et al., 2019).

Machine Learning in Education

Machine learning supports in learning to dyslexia peoples. Machine learning is computer program learned automatically from their experience. Basic concept of ML data is used to build or trains a model. Data used for building a model called training data (Reyana et al, 2020). ML makes generalization rules through observation of student domain knowledge and current performance. Computer based learning model uses machine learning approach to recognise student learning ability, predict performance of student, give feedback and take decision as teaching. It involves computer learning from data provided to carry out certain tasks.

OVERVIEW OF ASSISTIVE TECHNIQUES FOR DYSLEXICS

Dyslexia is phonological based problem occurs mostly in early age children. Early age intervention is needed to overcome this deficit. Most of the applications not provide immediate intervention even dyslexic children read incorrectly and they have need to aware about their mistakes and when help is needed. ASR provides immediate intervention. ASR technology not incorporate only target and correct words but also incorrect words read by children.

Recognition process takes user read speech as input and generates output. If output correct then continues reading otherwise immediate intervention is invoked, this allows user to inform mistake (Husni & Jamaludin, 2009). After feedback user asks for help button provided with application [5]. Data collected using samples of reading speech of children. Language examined results exhibits that most error made in vowel substitutions.

YUSR is an automatic speech recognition Arabic software for dyslexic children, analyze phonetic isolated of Arabic letters. Questionnaire, research and interviews conducted understand user needs (Schmidt & Schneider, 2007). YUSR provides two level interfaces to facilitate analyzing Arabic alphabet letters for dyslexics.

First level interface helps to learn and recognition of 28 Arabic alphabets for dyslexic children. By click on microphone icon, a child can record chosen letter pronunciation and get feedback. If child pronunciation accepted then congratulate feedback otherwise warning message to again pronounce (Taileb et al., 2013). Child listen correct pronunciation of letter by click on headphone icon and click on pencil icon to show how to write letter. The second interface listen pronunciation of a chosen letter to three positions at beginning, in middle and at last in words.

Mel-Frequency Cepstral Coefficients used for extracting features of sound for speech recognition. The Hidden Markov Model used for developing recognition process. More than 500 samples with different volume and sound of males and females used to trained application. The recognition rate 82% achieved by application.

Agent-DYSL system utilizes image processing and voice recognition to aid learner individual learning needs. The system goal is not only to inclusive learning materials but also to enhance reading skills with adapting and adjusting. Agent-DYSL allows adaptive assistance to dyslexic children to read text documents arbitrary, highlighting, emphasis on certain words. Vocabulary developed of the speech recognition module is based on reading errors. System vocabulary includes total 1321words of Greek language in which 1063 sentence words and 258 error sensitive words (Athanaselis et al., 2014). Recording and analysis component use image and speech recognition for data analysis. Knowledge infrastructure component provides learner's error profile. Profiling component used as store learner's error and preference of individual learner. Content presentation component receives PDF file then analysis of images and text and produce XML file.

Automatic speech recognition main goal is to record user voice when reads given text aloud and identifying reading errors, word mispronunciations, progress monitoring and user evaluation. By predicting reading errors Agent-DYSL intelligent system takes into account user profile update and user improvement. The module provides ability to process speech signal converting into a set of cepstral coefficients to perform feature extraction. Agent-DYSL system used by 23 children from 3rd to 5th grade in 6 public primary schools and 1 private center. After use of Agent-

DYSL the learner's reading pace increased by 0.52 units and 0.56 units after first and second evaluation respectively.

Reading accuracy of learner's also increased 0.56 units and 0.61 units after first and second evaluation respectively. Speech recognition performance improved using new algorithm and failure rate dropped by 36% to 21%.

For user evaluation and progress monitoring, the ASR will be able to recognize reading and detect user discrepancies from original text. The ASR enables the AGENT-DYSL reading system to predict user reading errors and also improvement users into account then update profile. The large vocabulary words both error-sensitive and sentence words in speech recognition engine based on Hidden Markov Models. The sensitive words selected based on visual confusion, composite, complex structure and stress words (Ouherrou et al. 2018).

An approach performing automatic transcription of read speech by dyslexic children using recognition engine trained on lexical and models. Automatic speech transcription facilitate to researchers by speech processing of recorded speech of dyslexic children. The system increase efficiency as compared to manual transcription which is very time consuming process. If transcription to large amount of dyslexic speech data, manual transcription tedious and extremely laborious. Automatic speech recognition engine perform tasks automatic labeling and transcribing speech into corresponding phonetics and textual representations, results in phoneme and text file of each read speech transcribed. Ten dyslexic children reading aloud and total 6112 speech samples are recorded in Malay (Husni, 2012). The preliminary result shows that automatic transcription approach provides 77% accuracy in phonetic labeling and transcriptions of dyslexic read speech.

Jollymate is notepad which recognizes handwritten character as correct or incorrect. It helps dyslexic students to do self learning. Children use this digital device improvement in the writing of letters. Lipi IDE is used as a character recognizer to identify the correctness of letters. The Child writes character on notepad and then input is sent to lipi toolkit after input processing of character making use of the processing module. By using neighbour classifier match input with training sample in lipi toolkit package, if the letter correctly matched then audio feedback and letter converted into a star. If a mismatch occurs audio feedback and open touch screen with assist letter practice. This device focuses on writing the practice of letters and improves learning skills (Khakhar & Madhvanath, 2010).

Dyseggxia is a mobile app dyslexia child to improve spelling skills with word exercise. The method is not to use correct words but to correct the exercise of wrong words used. Exercises were created using extract knowledge and error text written by dyslexia student through the realization of exercises to support the spelling (Rello et al., 2014). Development of games, apps, assistive technologies provides significant essential help to dyslexia children.

iLearnRW game following a personalized teaching programme for dyslexic student to improve their literacy skills. The aim of game design is to engagement of students, open-ended playing sessions with limited assets and literacy content. Play game outside of school hope to motivate students and improve learning outcomes, support to unsupervised effective learning and adaptation mechanism. iLearnRW consists of require students to exercise and repeat some activities regularly, towards gain accuracy and speed with respect to learning skills (Cuschieri et al. 2014).

LexiPal is learning model using gamification approach for dyslexic children incorporates 7 game elements. This model use windows presentation foundation technology to develop windows platform to create entertaining, enjoyment and

Table 1. Existing Assistive tools for dyslexic children

Software	Function	Tech.
Language tune-up kit	Software to teach reading to dyslexic children based on Orton-Gillingham method, teaches grammar, punctuations, and the rules	CD-ROM
Go phonics	Software to teach reading to dyslexic children based on Orton-Gillingham method, provides test and assessment	CD-ROM
Kurzweil 3000	Scan reading material and read out to them	TTS
TextHelp	Suggestion of spelling when typing, read aloud writing for checking	TTS
Clicker 4	Word processing support	TTS
Helpread	Read-along software while user are reading	TTS
Readplease	Read aloud text from web pages/emails	TTS
WordQ	Writing tool, suggest words, speech feedback	TTS
Via voice	Dictation software	ASR
Dragon naturally speaking	Dictation software	ASR
Mylexic	Dual coding theory, scaffolding teaching strategy, provide alphabet, syllables, word learning module	CD courseware
Dyslexia Baca	Confusion of letters by using Multisensory and Memorizing methods	Mobile app
iLearnRW	Student model by using machine leaning	Game software system
YUSR	Speech recognition, alphabet, phoneme based on HMM model of machine leaning	software
IASD	Phonological awareness, HMM model used	Standalone soft.
MyBaca	Sentence reading	courseware
E-Talk	Phoneme tone awareness	device
Jollymate	Multisensory learning using machine learning (k-NN &NN)	Digital notepad

motivation learning process. Gamification is basically used in game industry and studies, idea to insert game elements in non- game products such as education, commerce, health, work innovation, sharing, data gathering, intra-organizational systems and sustainable consumption (Kaur & Kautish, 2019). First goal is create interest and engagement of children with application. Evaluation of 40 dyslexic children describes they feel happy and enjoy when use application (Saputra & Risqi, 2015).

ANALYSIS OF DYSLEXIA ASSISTIVE TOOLS

Cause of dyslexia not measured scientifically. Functions and develops brain of a dyslexia person with different ways. Due to variation of disorder and ability between different dyslexics becomes quite challenging to assist all. Some simple recommendations Font Style, Formatting, Writing Style, size, colour, highlighted text and Layout ensure help to dyslexia children to reading.

For dyslexia have not direct solution, it can be managed or improve in learning through early intervention, methods, games, software's, mobile apps and under supervision of teachers, technicians who help to overcome disorders and give normal life. These technologies allowed new learning solutions for specialized education.

These games provides teaching learning environment which help in visual perception, memory development, time and space orientation, auditory ability, reasoning and motor coordination.

Majority of researchers have implemented ML models based techniques for dyslexic children to enhance their learning ability. Most of existing systems not fit according to expectations and limited their ability to use. So there is needs to a standardized system which provide novel features.

Some Currently available helping tools discussed mostly available in English, Malay, Arabic and some other languages. Assistive technique in Punjabi regional language for dyslexic is quite challenging task and main issues unaddressed till now thus opening a new research topic to develop assistive tool for dyslexic children in Punjabi language.

PROPOSED WORK

By keeping view of existing assistive techniques, so we have planned to effort towards building an assistive technique in Punjabi language which can be helpful for Punjabi dyslexics' children in their learning. Create a database of Punjabi Muharni pronounced by dyslexic children. Collect data of dyslexia children from different schools. Using an appropriate ML technique a model is designing and to develop an assistive technology. Evaluation of the proposed system results in higher accuracy and appropriate rate.

CONCLUSION

Automatic speech recognition is the key features to read dyslexics. ASR identifies dyslexic children making mistakes when reading and takes immediate intervention given as feedback. The application provides benefit to dyslexic children in reading by gives corrective feedback after incorrect reading. The accuracy of the recognition improved by read incorrect words into the vocabulary. ASR system enhances learning skills in dyslexic children. Such application provides useful and a suitable letter pronunciations for dyslexic children to encourage and improvement learning skills. Computer based techniques are very attractive to create interest in dyslexic children and motivate them to read with fun and excitement.

In future ASR application should also be develop in regional languages helping for dyslexic children in their own language. To improve traditional approaches an early intervention helping tool designed to assist dyslexia based on machine learning. It is diagnosed that early interventions in case of dyslexic children improve the learning style of these. Keeping all these points this paper proposes a system using machine learning technique which developed in future and helps for dyslexics.

REFERENCES

Athanaselis, T., Bakamidis, S., Dologlou, I., Argyriou, E. N., & Symvonis, A. (2011). Incorporating Speech Recognition Engine into an Intelligent Assistive Reading System for Dyslexic Students. *Twelfth Annual Conference of the International Speech Communication Association.*

Athanaselis, T., Bakamidis, S., Dologlou, I., Argyriou, E. N., & Symvonis, A. (2014). Making assistive reading tools user friendly: A new platform for Greek dyslexic students empowered by automatic speech recognition. *Multimedia Tools and Applications*, *68*(3), 681–699. doi:10.100711042-012-1073-5

Cuschieri, T., Khaled, R., Farrugia, V. E., Martinez, H. P., & Yannakakis, G. N. (2014, September). The iLearnRW game: support for students with Dyslexia in class and at home. In *2014 6th International Conference on Games and Virtual Worlds for Serious Applications (VS-GAMES)* (pp. 1-2). IEEE.

Elkind, J., Cohen, K., & Murray, C. (1993). Using computer-based readers to improve reading comprehension of students with dyslexia. *Annals of Dyslexia, 43*(1), 238–259. doi:10.1007/BF02928184 PMID:24233995

Hagen, A., Pellom, B., Van Vuuren, S., & Cole, R. (2004). Advances in children's speech recognition within an interactive literacy tutor. In *Proceedings of HLT-NAACL 2004: Short Papers* (pp. 25-28). 10.3115/1613984.1613991

Husni, H. (2012). Automatic transcription of dyslexic children-s read speech. *Global Journal on Technology*, 2.

Husni, H., & Jamaluddin, Z. (2008, October). A retrospective and future look at speech recognition applications in assisting children with reading disabilities. *Proceedings of the world Congress on Engineering and Computer Science.*

Husni, H., & Jamaludin, Z. (2009). ASR Technology for Children with Dyslexia: Enabling Immediate Intervention to Support Reading in Bahasa Melayu. *Online Submission, 6*(6), 64–70.

Islam, J., Mubassira, M., Islam, M. R., & Das, A. K. (2019, February). A speech recognition system for Bengali language using recurrent Neural network. In *2019 IEEE 4th international conference on computer and communication systems (ICCCS)* (pp. 73-76). IEEE.

Kaur, R., & Kautish, S. (2019). Multimodal sentiment analysis: A survey and comparison. *International Journal of Service Science, Management, Engineering, and Technology, 10*(2), 38–58. doi:10.4018/IJSSMET.2019040103

Khakhar, J., & Madhvanath, S. (2010, November). Jollymate: Assistive technology for young children with dyslexia. In *2010 12th International Conference on Frontiers in Handwriting Recognition* (pp. 576-580). IEEE.

Ouherrou, N., Elhammoumi, O., Benmarrakchi, F., & El Kafi, J. (2018, October). A heuristic evaluation of an educational game for children with dyslexia. In *2018 IEEE 5th International Congress on Information Science and Technology (CiSt)* (pp. 386-390). IEEE.

Rahman, F. A., Mokhtar, F., Alias, N. A., & Saleh, R. (2012). Multimedia elements as instructions for dyslexic children. *International Journal of Education and Information Technologies, 6*(2), 193–200.

Rani, S., & Kautish, S. (2018). Application of data mining techniques for prediction of diabetes-A review. International Journal of Scientific Research in Computer Science. *Engineering and Information Technology, 3*(3), 1996–2004.

Rani, S., & Kautish, S. (2018, June). Association clustering and time series based data mining in continuous data for diabetes prediction. In *2018 second international conference on intelligent computing and control systems (ICICCS)* (pp. 1209-1214). IEEE. 10.1109/ICCONS.2018.8662909

Raskind, M. H., & Higgins, E. L. (1999). Speaking to read: The effects of speech recognition technology on the reading and spelling performance of children with learning disabilities. *Annals of Dyslexia*, *49*(1), 251–281. doi:10.100711881-999-0026-9

Rello, L., Bayarri, C., Otal, Y., & Pielot, M. (2014, October). A computer-based method to improve the spelling of children with dyslexia. In *Proceedings of the 16th international ACM SIGACCESS conference on Computers & accessibility* (pp. 153-160). ACM.

Reyana, A., & Kautish, S. (2021). *Corona virus-related Disease Pandemic: A Review on Machine Learning Approaches and Treatment Trials on Diagnosed Population for Future Clinical Decision Support*. Current Medical Imaging.

Reyana, A., Krishnaprasath, V. T., Kautish, S., Panigrahi, R., & Shaik, M. (2020). Decision-making on the existence of soft exudates in diabetic retinopathy. *International Journal of Computer Applications in Technology*, *64*(4), 375–381. doi:10.1504/IJCAT.2020.112684

Russell, M., Brown, C., Skilling, A., Series, R., Wallace, J., Bonham, B., & Barker, P. (1996, October). Applications of automatic speech recognition to speech and language development in young children. In *Proceeding of Fourth International Conference on Spoken Language Processing. ICSLP'96* (Vol. 1, pp. 176-179). IEEE. 10.1109/ICSLP.1996.607069

Sampathkumar, A., Rastogi, R., Arukonda, S., Shankar, A., Kautish, S., & Sivaram, M. (2020). An efficient hybrid methodology for detection of cancer-causing gene using CSC for micro array data. *Journal of Ambient Intelligence and Humanized Computing*, *11*(11), 4743–4751. doi:10.100712652-020-01731-7

Saputra, M. R. U., & Risqi, M. (2015). LexiPal: Design, implementation and evaluation of gamification on learning application for dyslexia. *International Journal of Computers and Applications*, *131*(7), 37–43. doi:10.5120/ijca2015907416

Schmidt, A. P., & Schneider, M. (2007, September). Adaptive Reading Assistance for Dyslexic Students: Closing the Loop. In LWA (pp. 389-391). Academic Press.

Taileb, M., Al-Saggaf, R., Al-Ghamdi, A., Al-Zebaidi, M., & Al-Sahafi, S. (2013, July). YUSR: Speech recognition software for dyslexics. In *International Conference of Design, User Experience, and Usability* (pp. 296-303). Springer.

Williams, S. M., Nix, D., & Fairweather, P. (2013, April). Using speech recognition technology to enhance literacy instruction for emerging readers. In *Fourth International Conference of the Learning Sciences* (pp. 115-120). Academic Press.

Chapter 8
Mouse-Less Cursor Control for Quadriplegic and Autistic Patients Using Artificial Intelligence

Aman Sharma
Jaypee University of Information Technology, India

Saksham Chaturvedi
Jaypee University of Information Technology, India

ABSTRACT

Artificial intelligence is a field within computer science that attempts to simulate and build enhanced human intelligence into computers, mobiles, and various other machines. It can be termed as a powerful tool that has the capability to process huge sums of information with ease and assess patterns created over a period of time to give significant results or suggestions. It has garnered focus from almost every field from education to healthcare. Broadly, AI applications in healthcare include early detection and diagnosis, suggesting treatments, evaluating progress, medical history, and predicting outcomes. This chapter discussed AI, ASD, and what role AI currently plays in advancing autistic lives including detection, analysis, and treatment of ASD and how AI has been improving healthcare and the existing medical and technology aids available for autistic people. Current and future advancements are discussed and suggested in the direction of improving social abilities and reducing the communication and motor difficulties faced by people with ASD.

DOI: 10.4018/978-1-7998-7460-7.ch008

INTRODUCTION

Autism Spectrum Disorder is a lifelong neurological developmental disorder characterised by repetitive patterns of behaviour and impaired development in communication, interaction, and understanding of social clues. Genes also play a significant role in the increasing number of cases of ASD as it can be inherited genetically. It is called a spectrum disorder because of the wide variation in the type and severity of symptoms experienced by autistic individuals. They suffer from verbal and non-verbal communication impairments, motor difficulties and have limited range of interests and activities. They find it difficult to communicate with people, spontaneously greet them, understand facial expressions, maintain eye contact and perform decision making. Some of them face difficulty in grasping or manipulating objects, such as a ball or a mouse. Inability to use the mouse continually for hours makes it difficult for them to use computers and perform even the simple tasks on it.

AI has shown confident results in fields of engineering, surveillance, business, healthcare and everyday applications using its models of Deep Learning, Machine Learning, Neural Networks and their applications including image recognition, large data set analysis, speech recognition, biometric verification, chatbots, natural language generation, sentiment analysis and more. Broadly, AI applications in healthcare include early detection & diagnosis, suggesting treatments, evaluating progress, medical history and predicting outcomes. Hence, increasing efforts are being made to incorporate AI into lesser researched or detailed healthcare sectors like Autism. AI-driven approaches help in developing predictive models by utilizing the hidden correlations and patterns in the data. Currently, the most prevalent use of AI for autistic individuals includes

1. Robots and Web or Mobile Applications; to teach the children and improve their interaction and communication abilities.
2. Assistance to therapists and doctors by analysing and assessing a child's videos and reports.
3. Mobile Applications to provide mental health support to autistic children as well as to make people conscious of autistic people's needs.

The responsibility of diagnosis, treatment and progress evaluation of an autistic individual on the therapists and, further care taken by parents or care takers could be reduced with the help of humanoid robots and virtual assistants. Autistic children find it comparatively easier to interact with robots than humans as robots are less complex than humans and also provide them a similar feeling as that of playing with toys.

The chapter is majorly focused on introducing "Mouse-less Cursor Control" technology as a way out

1. To proceed in the direction of reducing the challenges faced by autistic children and similar people due to communication & motor impairments,
2. To make aforesaid people more self-reliant and self-sufficient,
3. To provide them ease in performing work & communication at the office or at home via computer/laptop with the help of AI-based innovations.

Information related to a demo model to imitate and test the "Mouse-less Cursor Control" using facial movements is also discussed. It is a Human Computer Interaction application which uses Python and its libraries including Numpy, OpenCV, PyAuto GUI, Dlib and Imutils to work. Commercial products such as Smyle Mouse, Ishara and more, which are already available in the market working upon the same technology, are also mentioned.

BACKGROUND

Various studies have highlighted the use of artificial intelligence in the healthcare industry. AI-based tools have improved diagnostics, treatment guidance, feedbacks, prognosis and patient outcomes. It is also evident that in the future, AI will become an integral part of the healthcare services. According to Sixty-Seventh World Health Assembly Geneva (2014, May), Autism Spectrum Disorder is a developmental disorder that emerges in early childhood and persists throughout the lifespan of most individuals. They experience impaired development in social interaction, communication and have a limited skill sets and interest in activities. The challenges they come across include social stigma and disapprobation, mood instability, isolation, discrimination, and many do not have access to proper medical support and services (Kaur & Kautish, 2019). The initial assessment costs for ASD may range from $700 to $2,000 (Katie Parsons, 2018) and a therapy treatment costs around $1200 per week, which can continue for years depending on the child's need. Depending on whether the autistic child has any co-occurring intellectual disabilities or not, their education, health, and other service needs can cost from $1.4 and upto $2.4 million dollars (Buescher AV, Cidav Z et al., 2014). The numbers may vary depending upon family's lifestyle, extent of care that the individual requires, range and severity of symptoms etc. The treatments or therapies are devised according to every child's unique needs as ASD is a spectrum disorder and one solution will not work for every child. It requires an expert clinician's careful observation and frequent evaluation of the child's behaviour.

Since intervention should begin as early as possible, AI may help (Sampathkumar et al 2020) not only in the early diagnosis of ASD but also in the therapy process by helping in improving their communication abilities, learn developmental skills, reduce harmful behaviours including self-injury and aggressive behaviour towards other people. According to Indian Academy of Pediatrics (Dr. SS Kamath, Dr Samir Dalwai, 2017), children should be screened with standardized autism screening tool between 18 months and 2 years of age. Figure 1 explains the flow of developmental screening activities (Centers for Disease Control and Prevention 2020, Feb). However, due to limited health professionals and infrastructure many children are diagnosed years later. Recently, socially-assistive robots have introduced more affordable and personalized care. It might help in reducing the excess demand for therapy services and the burden on the therapists to facilitate everything, from diagnosis to learning.

Figure 1. Pediatric Developmental Screening flowchart
(Centers for Disease Control and Prevention 2020, Feb)

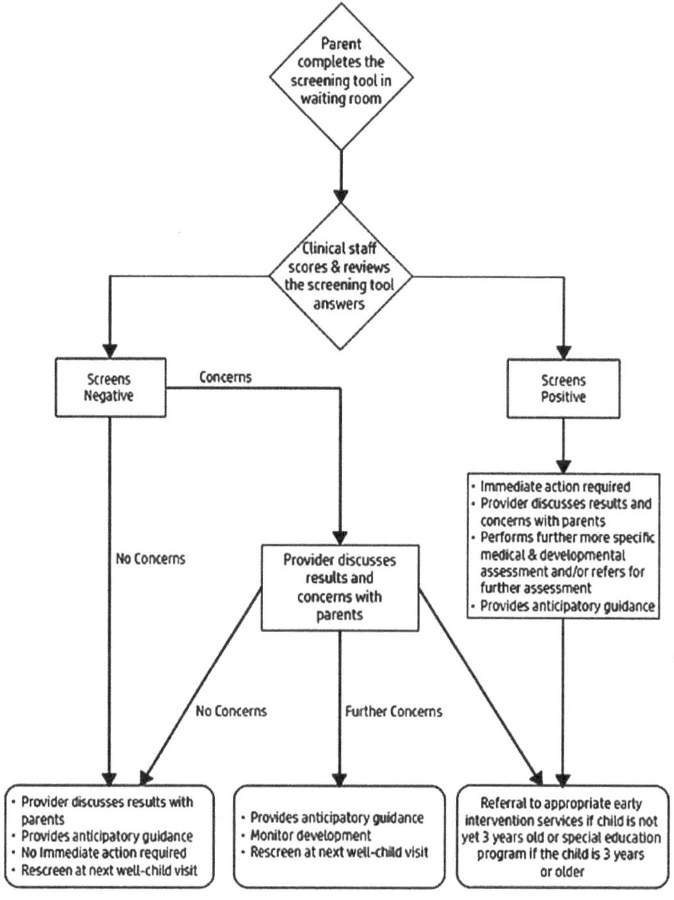

Figure 2. Majorly observed symptoms of ASD

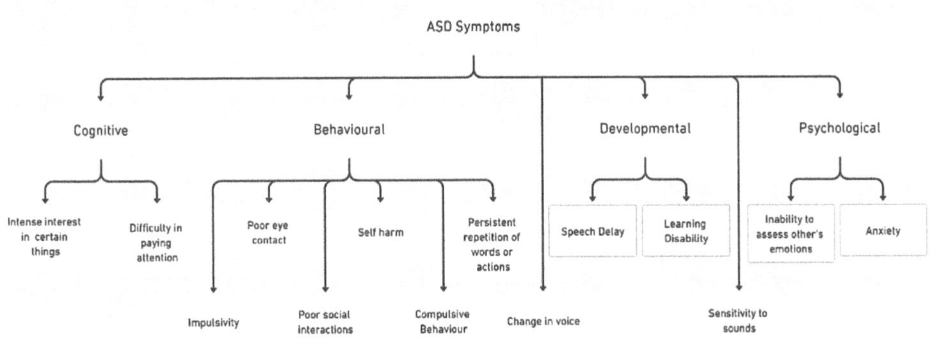

ASD SYMPTOMS

Earliest symptoms of ASD include absence of normal behaviour. Some of the typical symptoms and signs used by therapists to judge are explained in Figure 2.

ASD being a heterogeneous neuro developmental disorder, the cause, the aetiology and the genetic landscape of it remains unknown. It is termed as a spectrum disorder (Rani, & Kautish, 2018) because of the wide variation in the type and severity of symptoms experienced by autistic individuals and so, it is not necessary that an autistic child will experience all of the above discussed symptoms. Cases of ASD have been increasing widely from one generation to another all over the world as it can be inherited from the parents. So, developing a clear picture of exactly what ASD is and its treatments, is increasingly becoming crucial.

Motor Difficulties Faced by Autistic, Quadriplegics and Other Individuals

ASD appears to have a vivid increase over the last couple of years; 87% of autistic people according to a recent estimate (Lauren Schenkman, 2020) have some sort of motor difficulty but, it is not considered as a core trait of Autism because they also occur with other conditions, such as Quadriplegia, Cerebral Palsy, Arthritis and Attention Deficit Hyperactivity Disorder (ADHD). Some of the disorders/diseases related to motor difficulties are listed in Table 1.

Some common motor difficulties between Autistic individuals and some discussed above include:

1. Poor fine-motor control
    a. Causes difficulty in manipulating objects and writing.

2. Gross-motor problems
    a. Clumsy, uncoordinated gait.
3. Poorly coordinated movements between the left and right side of the body among different limbs.
4. Trouble with actions requiring hand-eye coordination, such as grasping objects, catching a ball, writing sentences or imitating the movements.

The motor difficulties discussed above cause hindrance to using computers for a long time as grasping, clicking, continually hovering the mouse and typing becomes extremely exhaustive. Also, trying to hide or masking the inability or anxiety can add up to the fatigue and may lead to overexertion (National Autistic Society, 2020). It is not necessary that all autistic people face the discussed motor disabilities as Autism is a spectrum disorder and its symptoms can be different for every child.

Instant Captions with Speech Recognition Technology can be used as an alternative to actual typing on the keyboard. But the need for an alternate solution for the mouse is still there.

Table 1. List of disorders

S No.	Disorder/Disease	Details
1	Quadriplegia	Paralysis caused due to illness or injury resulting in the partial or total loss of use of all four limbs and torso.
		Loss of sensation and control.
2	Cerebral palsy	Brain injury which causes a decrease in muscle control.
		Interferes with dexterity in using a mouse.
3	Muscular Dystrophy	Genetic disorder.
		Abnormal genes (mutations) lead to muscle degeneration.
4	Hand Arthritis	Affects joints of the hands causing swelling and stiffness.
		Causes pain with movement or when at rest.
5	Multiple Sclerosis	Immune disease that attacks the central nervous system.
		Causes communication problems between brain and rest of the body.
		Many experience numbness in arms and hands.
6	Stroke	Ruptured/blocked blood vessels in brain which cause interruption in oxygen & blood supply to the brain.
		Causes muscle fatigue
7	Cleft Hand	Parts of fingers in the center of the hand are missing.
		Usually V-shaped hands
		Lack of fingers causes problems in manipulating and grasping objects.

Although, the above discussed disorders are very different from each other, a common strategy can be adopted for providing ease in using computer and performing even the simplest tasks like web-surfing by replacing the traditional mouse with a "Mouse-less Cursor Control" technology.

DRUGS AND AUTISM

Non-drug therapies, which include psychology-based therapy like cognitive behaviour therapy (Reyana, & Kautish, 2021), positive behaviour encouragement, social skills training and sensory integration therapy, are primarily considered for the treatment of ASD. Drug treatment is not considered as effective as non-drug therapies for the core symptoms of Autism but they may have a role in managing comorbidities and related symptoms (Sharma, S. R. et al., 2018), such as irritability and aggression. For assistance in managing aggression and irritable behaviours, risperidone or aripiprazole may be used, according to the most research-based data at present.

According to studies performed during 1950s and 1960s, it was considered that autism represented a childhood version of adult psychosis or schizophrenia and the treatment was done according to the clinical psychiatry of that time (Eisenberg, L., 1957). In the early 1960s, psychiatric treatments including electroshock therapy, insulin shock, amphetamines, and antidepressants were used to help children with autism (Bender L., Goldschmidt L. et al., 1962). In between 1959 and 1974, researchers administered the use of a psychedelic drug, LSD (Sigafoos, J., et al., 2007), as an experimental therapy for the treatment of children with autism probably to curb the most common comorbidities with autism i.e. depression and anxiety. Researches are being conducted on the use of LSD in healthcare for therapeutic purposes but it is not recommended for the treatment of autism yet.

People with autism generally tend to interpret neutral facial expressions negatively (Soichiro Matsuda, et al., 2015) for which, according to anecdotal reports, MDMA drug might help in improving their ability to assess more accurately and, as a consequence, become less socially inhibited. This is so as the effects of MDMA drug include an enhanced sense of well-being and increased extroversion due to greater production of serotonin, dopamine, and norepinephrine than usual. But it could also possess risk of decreasing the already hampered ability to interpret fear or anxiety in others as currently there are no FDA-approved pharmacological treatments available for autistic people with social anxiety, and the conventional anti-anxiety medications lack clinical effectiveness for them.

HOW COMPUTERS AND AI CAN HELP AUTISTIC PEOPLE?

Autism's early diagnosis is crucial to come up with effective early interventions. Along with it more initiatives are required to ease their lives since Autism is a lifelong condition and like other normal human beings, they also need to make a living and live peacefully and happily. There are many autistic people who are unable to acquire jobs but many of those who do get jobs, feel underemployed. Computers and laptops have become an integral part of human life now and unlike earlier, the need for humans to do the heavy physical work has decreased to a large extent as most of the work is done using computers and other machinery. Although not for the roles that require considerable interaction with other people such as an HR and sales, knowing how to use a computer and using it effectively can land them at least somewhere to work, from being a journalist to a computer programmer or a software developer.

Even after intensive therapy treatments (Reyana et al, 2020), it remains unclear of what and how the autistic child is feeling. It is observed that autistic children have a better relation with computers than human in terms of interest and interaction because computers or robots are not as complex as humans when it comes to emotional communication and they provide them similar feeling as that of playing with toys. Computers can allow autistic people to express their feelings and communicate by typing to it as it did for Carly, allowing to express herself in words for the first time in her life (ABC News, 2012).

Children who wish to write, but cannot because of inability in manipulating and grasping objects, can make use of technologies like live-transcribing. AI enabled live transcribing applications help in providing Instant Captions with Speech Recognition Technology.

For leisure activities, the person can enjoy the company of a virtual assistant like Google Assistant, Siri etc.

An autistic child may have deep interest in a certain topic. Since they might not be very comfortable in interacting with a human teacher in person to learn about their interests, they can opt for the mode of online learning. Online Learning platforms are better suited for them as they provide a sense of controlled environment which helps them curb their anxiety. Many extend their interests in software development as programming is an engaging activity plus, it provides a sense of control over the code i.e. they can control how and what they want to create by typing the appropriate commands.

But, for them to be able to perform tasks on a laptop or a computer, methods that require the least amount of physical efforts are needed to be devised.

MOUSE-LESS CURSOR CONTROL USING FACIAL MOVEMENTS

Mouse-less Cursor Control using Facial Movements is an effort to remove people's dependency on the hardware including a mouse and a keyboard, to be able to interact with the computer. This could be done using the knowledge of Human-Computer Interaction. HCI is a multidisciplinary field of study that focuses on improving the interaction between humans and computers and also studies the design, execution and assessment of computer systems. It is concerned with making systems easy to learn and use. The "Mouse-less Cursor Control using Facial Movements" is an example of an HCI (Human-Computer Interaction) application which allows the user to control the mouse cursor with its facial movements. The model works by predicting the facial landmarks of a given face. From facial landmarks, eye blinks (Adrian Rosebrock, 2017), mouth and nose movements (Adrian Rosebrock, 2017) can be detected to trigger designed actions.

Existing literature (Kaur, Kanwaljit & Pany, et al. (2017), Ramdoss, S. et al. (2011), Smith V., et al. (2014)) supports the effectiveness of computer-based interventions in reducing the cognitive, communication, and social disabilities dealt by autistic individuals. Alongside the ongoing research on diagnosis and treatment of ASD using AI, HCI is used for mediating communication and development of emotional skills (Constain Moreno, et al., 2018).

Requirements

1. Computer or Laptop
2. Webcam

A basic model (Akshay L Chandra, 2018) for the discussed utility can be created by anyone with a-little prior coding knowledge as it requires understanding of the language- Python (Mihajlović et al., 2020) and its libraries. Python is the most preferred language for developing artificial intelligence solutions.

Advantages of using Python for AI include:

- Access to numerous libraries and frameworks for AI
    - TensorFlow: for machine learning workloads and working with datasets.
    - Scikit-learn: provides tools including regression, classification, clustering, model selection, processing for modeling data.
    - Pybrain: offers powerful machine learning algorithms.
- Simplicity
    - The concise and readable code of Python makes it easier to use.

- Less Code
    - Least efforts in coding are required with Python when compared to other languages.
- Platform independence & Flexibility
    - It enables developers to use it on multiple platforms like Windows, Linux, macOS etc. Minimal changes are required to migrate the source code.
- Wide community
    - It has huge community support from users worldwide.
    - Helpful when there comes any coding error to address.

Libraries which may be used along with Python for the discussed utility include:

- Numpy
    - As working with arrays is faster than lists.
    - Arrays help in holding more than one value at a time under a single name.
    - Better loading, manipulating and summarizing of data.
- OpenCV
    - Provides optimised machine learning algorithms for computer vision applications.
    - Enables real-time vision, facial recognition, object detection using classic, advance computer vision and machine learning algorithms.
    - Popular application: Google's self-driving car.
- PyAutoGUI
    - Provides cross-platform GUI automation.
    - The top left corner of the screen is denoted as the (0, 0) origin and while the x-coordinates increase going rightwards, the y coordinates increase going downwards.
    - Used to move the mouse-cursor according to the head or nose movement.
- Imutils
    - Includes basic image processing functions such as detecting edges, translation and more.
    - Implemented along with OpenCV and Python.
- Dlib
    - Toolkit containing machine learning algorithms and tools for creating complex software in C++ to solve real world problems.
    - Dlib's shape predictor file is used as a trained model for estimating facial landmarks.

Prebuilt Model Details

The model requires two important functions.

1. A detector to detect the face
2. A predictor to predict the facial landmarks.

The Histogram of Oriented Gradients (HOG) feature combined with a linear classifier, an image pyramid, and sliding window detection scheme can be used for the face detector while for the facial landmarks estimator regression approach can be taken (Kazemi, V., & Sullivan, J., 2014). Some of the face detection methods using OpenCV and Dlib are discussed in Table 2.

Out of the above discussed methods, according to the source (Akshay L Chandra, 2018), HOG classifier using Dlib is considered for face detection. Working of HOG is shown in figure 3.

Figure 3. Working of HOG

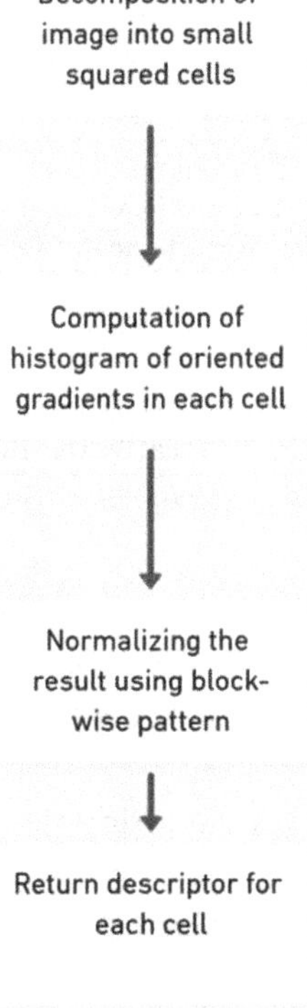

Table 2. Different Face Detection methods in OpenCV and Dlib

S No.	Models	Characteristics	Details
1	**HAAR Cascade**	Platform	OpenCV
		Pros	1. Ability to run almost real-time on CPU 2. Simple architecture 3. Ability to detect faces across different scales
		Cons	1. False predictions 2. Poor performance with non-frontal images 3. Doesn't work under occlusion
2	**DNN Face Detector**	Platform	OpenCV, Deep Learning
		Pros	1. Accuracy 2. Ability to run at real-time on CPU 3. Works with different face orientations 4. Ability to detect difference in face sizes 5. Works under substantial occlusion)
		Cons	1. Slower than HOG face detector
3	**HOG Face Detector**	Platform	Dlib
		Pros	1. Fastest method on CPU (among the discussed) 2. Detects slightly non-frontal faces also 3. Works under small occlusion 4. Light-weight model
		Cons	1. Does not detect small faces as it is trained for minimum face size of 80×80 2. The bounding box often excludes part of forehead and chin 3. Poor performance with non-frontal faces 4. Does not work under substantial occlusion
4	**CNN Face Detector**	Platform	Dlib, Deep Learning
		Pros	1. Detects different face orientations 2. Easy training process 3. Works under occlusion
		Cons	1. Poor performance on CPU 2. Does not detect small faces as it is trained for minimum face size of 80×80 3. The bounding box often excludes part of forehead and chin, is even smaller than the HOG detector.

In a study similar to mouse-less cursor control (Singh, A., Chandewar, C. et al., 2018), HOG classifier and HAAR methods are compared in which HOG method is considered over the HAAR because of the following reasons:

1. HOG features are capable of capturing the user's outline/shape better than HAAR features.
2. HAAR cascade classifier is affected by the variation in light intensity. If an object has HAAR wavelets similar to that of a face, it recognizes that object as a face.

3. HOG classifier works on the principal of segmentation and hence perfectly detects profile face and the 68 facial landmarks.

A trained model for processing high quality face recognition can be obtained from the Dlib library under the image processing section (Dlib C++ Library, List of files). Note that the model file used in (Akshay L Chandra, 2018) expects the bounding boxes from the face detector to be aligned according to the Dlib's HOG face detector and will not work properly with a face detector that produces boxes in a different alignment, such as the CNN based "mmod_human_face_detector.dat" face detector.

Facial Landmark Estimator

Facial landmark detection is used to detect the key landmarks on the face and obtain an understanding of the face shape. It has many uses in the field of computer vision and plays a major role in 3D face reconstruction (Asthana, A., et al. (2011), Hu, Y. et al., 2004), face animation- in-app filters (Cao, C. et al. 2014) and face recognition (Huang, G. B. et al. (2014), Berg, T. et al. (2012), Zhu, X. et al. (2015)).

With time, the need for more clear and accurate identification of facial landmarks has increased. Regression-based algorithms are preferred over methods that use parameterized models to describe the face shape and appearance (Cootes, T. F. et al.(1995), T. F. Cootes et al.(2001), Zhu, X. et al.(2012)). Methods for regression-based facial landmark detection usually learn a series of mapping and regression functions to progressively update the estimated landmark positions towards the actual locations. A high-performance landmark detection algorithm includes the pose-indexed robust features (Dollár, P. et al. 2010), the cascade regression structure (Cao, X. et al. 2014), and the regression model (Xiong, X. et al.(2013), Ren, S. et al. (2016), Kazemi, V., & Sullivan, J. (2014)).

Landmark localization for geometric face normalization can be used for improving the recognition results by recognizing the facial movements efficiently and hence triggering the supposed actions.

For detecting eye blinks from a standard/inbuilt webcam, a real-time algorithm is required. A support vector machine classifier helps in detecting eye blinks as a pattern of eye-aspect-ratio values in a short temporal window (Sagonas, C., Antonakos et al. 2016).

Along with eyes and eyebrows, other facial regions including nose, mouth, jaw can be extracted using Dlib's pre-trained facial landmark detector (Adrian Rosebrock, 2017).

Figure 4. Landmark configurations of different databases
(Sagonas, C., Antonakos et al. 2016)

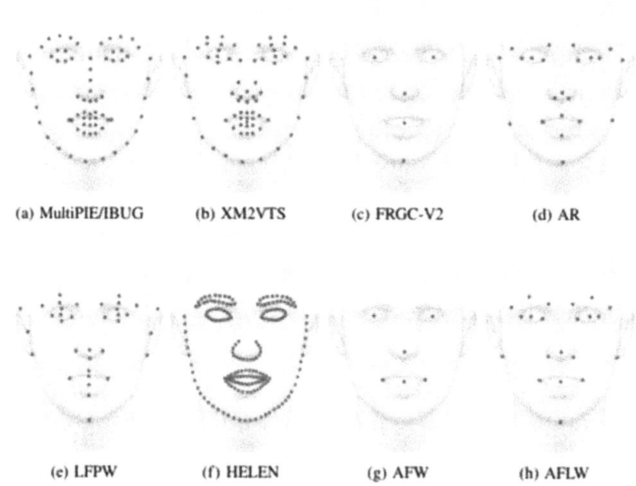

Dataset

The iBUG 300 dataset is a semi-automatic annotation methodology for annotating massive face datasets. It contains 50 "in-the-wild" videos, mostly recorded from a TV, in which each frame has a precise annotation of the facial landmarks (Sagonas, C., Antonakos et al. (2016), (2013), (2013)). It uses a 68 points mark-up for the annotations as shown in Figure 5.

The license for this dataset however does not permit commercial use and therefore, the trained model cannot be used in a commercial product.

Working and Methodology

A basic model can be created to try and understand the working of a mouse-less cursor using facial movements with the help of the programming language, Python, the aforementioned libraries and a training dataset (Akshay L Chandra, 2018). Figure 6 shows the working process for a basic model in a simplified manner,

1. Facial Landmarks Are Predicted

Facial landmarks are used to calculate further required components (EAR, MAR) and then trigger the functions to control the mouse cursor using facial movements. Detection and extraction of facial landmarks is done using Dlib, OpenCV.

Figure 5. The 68 facial coordinate points (iBUG 300-W dataset)
(Sagonas, C., Antonakos et al. 2016)

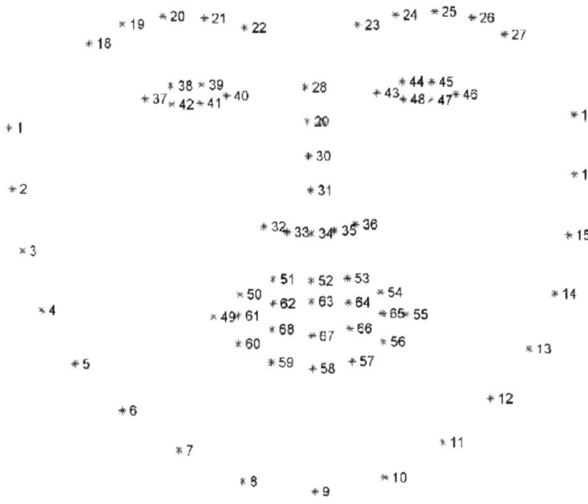

Figure 6. Working process of a basic model for controlling mouse cursor with facial movements

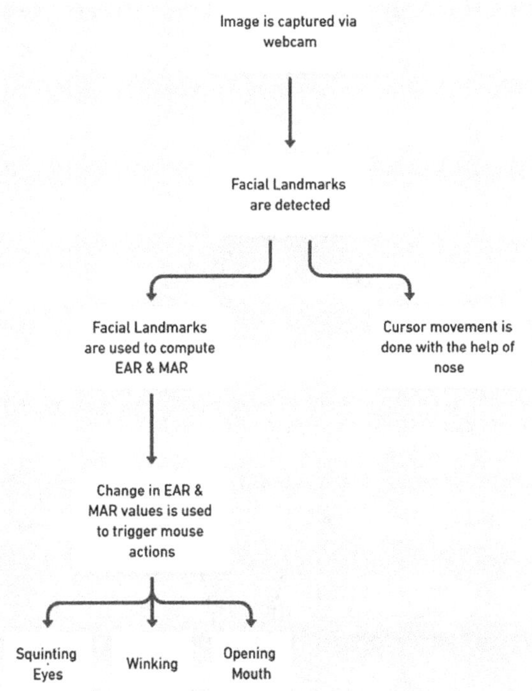

2. Eye-Aspect -Ratio (EAR) Is Calculated

- EAR can be defined as an estimate of the eye-opening state. Traditional image processing methods for computing blinks involve eye localization (Hockey, G. R. J. et al. 2003), thresholding to find the whites of the eyes (Lefkovits, S. et al. 2017) and determining if the "white" region of the eyes disappears for a period, indicating a blink (Fernández, A. et al. 2016). Eye aspect ratio metric is preferred as it provides real time eye-blink detection (Soukupova, T., & Cech, J., 2016).
- The ratio is computed between height and width of the eye where points "p1" to "p6" are the 2D landmark locations as depicted in figure 7. The formula for calculating EAR is

$$\frac{|| p2 - p6 || + || p3 - p5 ||}{2 || p1 - p4 ||}.$$

The EAR calculated of both eyes is averaged as the eyes blink simultaneously.

- The EAR value changes upon the extent of opening and closing of the eyes. It increases on opening and decreases on closing of the eyes.
- The EAR value is mostly constant when the eyes are open and it gets closer to zero as the eyes tend to close. Figure 8 shows the variation in EAR as eyes open and close.

Figure 7. EAR landmarks

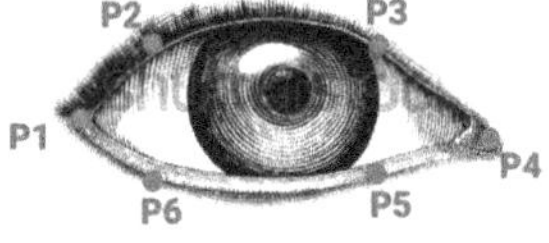

Figure 8. Variation in EAR with eyes opening and closing
(Singh, A., Chandewar, C. et al. 2018)

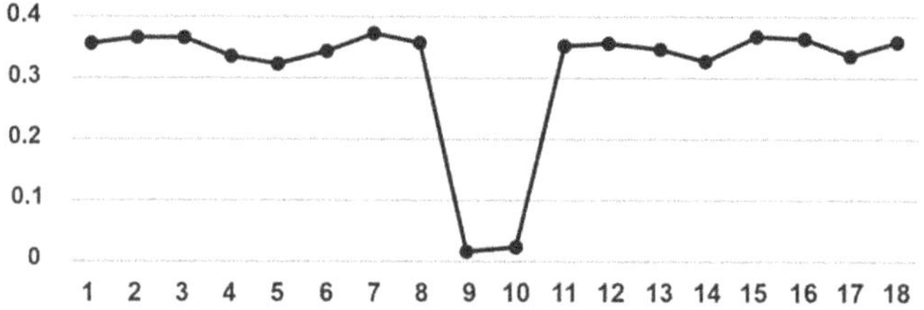

3. Mouth-Aspect Ratio (MAR) Is Calculated

Similar to the EAR,

- MAR is the ratio computed between height and width of the mouth where points "p1" to "p8" are the 2D landmark locations as depicted in figure 9. The formula for calculating MAR is

$$\frac{\| p2 - p8 \| + \| p3 - p7 \| + \| p4 - p6 \|}{2 \| p1 - p5 \|}.$$

- As the mouth is opened, the MAR value increases and as it is closed, the MAR value tends to zero as shown in Figure 10.

4. Actions That Act as Triggers to Control the Mouse

- Nose/Head movement
  - To manoeuvre the cursor.
  - Head movements may include yaw, pitch and diagonal.

Figure 9. MAR landmarks

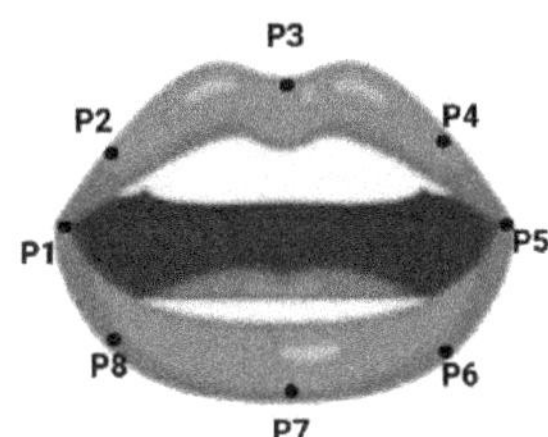

Figure 10. Variation of MAR with mouth opening and closing
(Singh, A., Chandewar, C. et al. 2018)

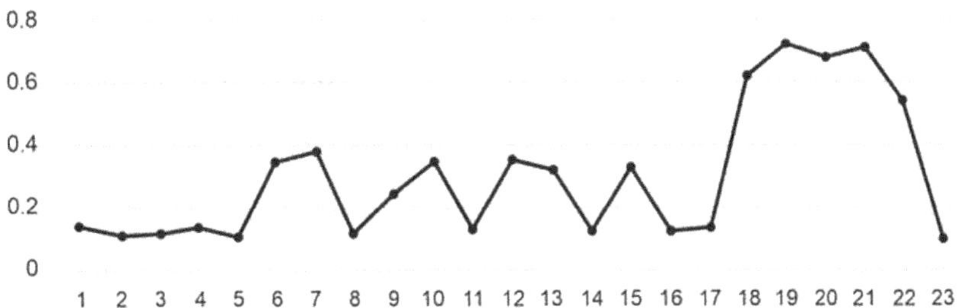

- Opening of mouth
    - To activate cursor or scrolling.
- Eye blinks
    - to click Right/ Left.

COMMERCIALLY AVAILABLE PRODUCTS BASED ON THE CONCEPT- MOUSE-LESS CURSOR CONTROL USING FACIAL MOVEMENTS

- **Ishara:** 'Ishara' is a perceptive user interface that (Saikat Basak, 2017), similar to having control over a cursor with facial movements, offers control via hand gestures and requires the built-in computer camera or USB webcam and its software.
    - The camera is placed such that it faces the user and with the help of two different colour-markers on the fingers, the mouse pointer is controlled.
    - Available actions include left/right click, scroll and drag-and-drop.

This utility might be useful for some of the autistic people but not for those who cannot manoeuvre their hands and fingers so efficiently or those who experience fatigue in a little time of action.

- **Animouse:** Animouse is a free and open-source software which tracks the user's head movements with the computer's webcam to control the mouse cursor (Aniket Eknath Kudale, 2015). It is only Windows operating system compatible.
- **Smyle Mouse:** Smyle Mouse is a commercially available product for hands-free computer control (Smyle Mouse, https://smylemouse.com/).
    - It works by capturing the facial gestures through the webcam or the inbuilt camera.
    - It requires the user to move their head to move the pointer and smile to perform a click or make an adaptive switch selection.
    - It is designed for Microsoft Windows 7/8/10 operating system only.
- **HeadMouse:** HeadMouse is another commercially available product that converts a user's head movements into the mouse pointer movement (Origin Instruments, *HeadMouse®*).
    - Head Mouse Nano provides webcam hardware for high resolution tracking and pixel-precise control over the cursor & gets connected to the device via USB.

    - It has a wireless optical sensor which tracks a tiny disposable target that the user wears on their forehead, glasses, or hat to control the pointer.
    - It can connect to any device that supports a USB port, and operates using standard mouse drivers. It does not require a special software as it is powered by the host device, over the USB connection.
- **Enable Viacam:** Enable Viacam (eViacam) is a free, open-source mouse replacement software that allows the user to control their computer mouse with their head movements (Enable Viacam, https://eviacam.crea-si.com/index.php).
    - It works on any standard computer equipped with a webcam and similar to other discussed products, does not require additional hardware.
- **EVA Facial Mouse:** EVA Facial Mouse is an Android mobile application (available on Google Play, CREA Software Systems- EVA Facial Mouse PRO) that tracks the user's face using artificial vision techniques and allows the user to control the device according to the facial movements captured through the front camera.
    - The pointer on the screen allows access to the interface elements and is controlled by the user's head movements.
    - An on-screen menu enables to choose the desired gesture or action to perform, like scroll, swipe etc.
    - Some limitations include:
        - Lack of support for most games.
        - Difficult to use with smaller screen-sized device.
        - Applications that require access to the camera cannot be used simultaneously.
        - Applications including Google Maps, Google Earth and Gallery work with restrictions.

LIMITATIONS OF THE MOUSE-LESS CURSOR CONTROL USING FACIAL MOVEMENTS

The discussed, currently-basic model of the "Mouse-less Cursor Control using Face Movements" has some challenges to overcome including:

- The program (Akshay L Chandra, 2018) is not very smooth and also not optimized enough for production or commercial use and full-fledged incorporation into computer systems. It can be used as a demo to understand the working of the commercially available products which exercise similar idea and technology.

- The actions are not public-friendly i.e., working while winking and opening mouth might seem weird to do in public.
- The trigger actions are limited and may cause difficulty to some people like patients of benign-positional-vertigo who experience a sudden mild or intense sensation of their head spinning due to change in the head's positioning, however, the symptoms generally last for less than a minute (Fernández, A., Usamentiaga, et al. 2016).
- Many old-age people might not be able to perform the actions.

CURRENT AI DEVELOPMENTS AND LIMITATIONS

AI is not one technology, and has many subsets. Figure 11 lists some of the categories of AI which play high importance in healthcare.

(Davenport, T., & Kalakota, R., 2019) Machine Learning is a technique by which data models are created and trained to perform tasks accordingly. In the healthcare sector, it helps in suggesting the medicines and treatments protocols to be followed for optimum results according to the details provided by the patient. It does so by analysing large data sets and judging the symptoms with the help of its pre-trained models. Figure 12 describes the general methodology for machine learning applications.

Neural Network technology helps in determining whether a patient will acquire a particular disease. Neutral network models along with deep learning help in predicting outcomes (Fakoor, Rasool et al. 2013). The combination helps in providing greater accuracy in diagnosis, speech recognition (Natural Language Processing) and image-analysis. This attribute of AI is also used to provide assistance to autistic individuals in using computers.

Natural Language Processing, in healthcare, is mostly used for creation, classification and analysis of the clinical reports of patients. It has been noticed that often times some things remain unclear between the autistic children and the therapist due to inefficient communication and attributes like avoiding eye-contact

Figure 11. Types of AI of major relevance to healthcare

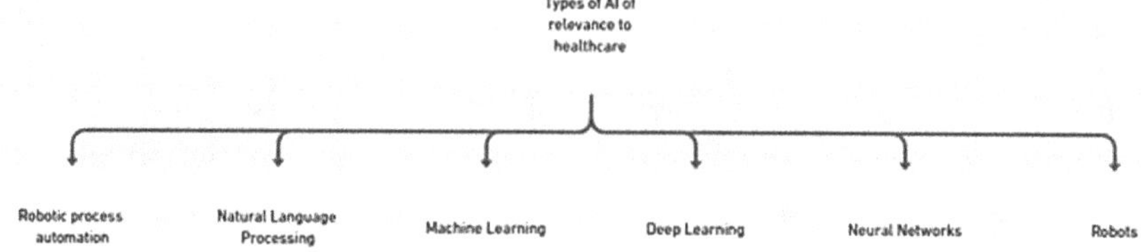

Figure 12. General methodology for machine learning applications

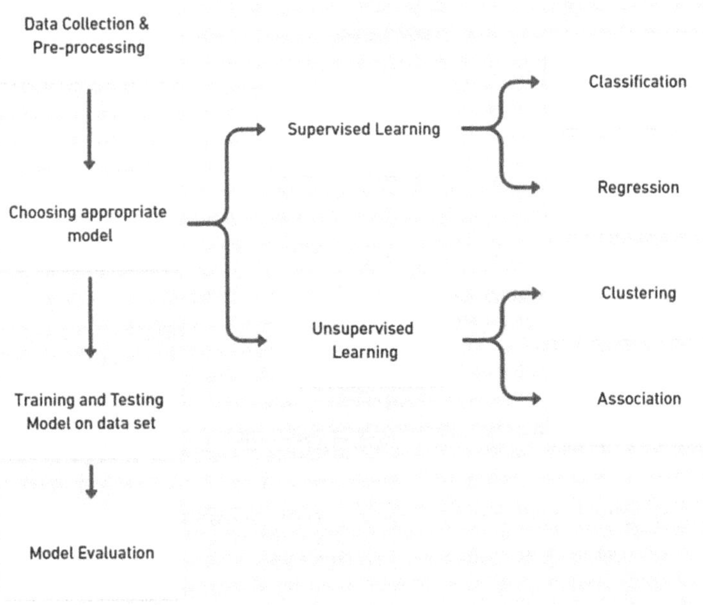

by the child. Some sources have stated that autistic children seemed to be more comfortable communicating to AI-robots because then they did not feel uninterested in relating with the robot or stressed or negative about making eye-contact. NLP can help transcribe patient interactions which could be later assessed by the therapist.

Robotic process automation, unlike other forms of AI, requires minimal investment, has low technical barrier i.e. it is easy to implement and is extremely accurate. Robotic process automation does not involve physical robots but only computer servers. It helps in performing repetitive tasks like updating patient records and billing.

Use of physical robots is prevalent in many industries including healthcare like providing surgical precision and their use as exoskeletons. They help by performing the tasks pre-defined to them like, lifting and repositioning things, delivering supplies in hospitals. AI capabilities of the robots has enabled them to learn things over-time.

All the above discussed technologies can be used collectively to achieve better solutions.

AI, Robots and Applications Aiding Autism

Several robots including Keepon (Kozima, H. et al. 2009), Hanson Robokind (Hanson, D. et al.2012), Bandit (Duquette et al.2008), and Kaspar (J. Wainer et al.2014) are helping autistic children develop their social interaction and communication skills.

Nao (Tapus et al.2012), a humanoid robot, uses its two 2D cameras and four directional microphones to record the child's facial expressions and body language as they interact and carefully assesses the data to gain the child's attention and keep them engaged in interaction.

Robots can be excellent tutors also, in terms of their ability to repeat instructions and interact constantly without getting tired. According to studies, they have been successful in showing an increase in some of the autistic children's social interaction and communication abilities (Jason Falconer, IEEE Spectrum, 2013).

Robokind's Milo (Abrams et al.(2018), Robokind (n.d.)) is another humanoid robot that uses "Applied Behaviour Analysis" therapy to teach social skills to children with autism and also provide them immediate feedback about their responses. Its ability to show emotions through facial expressions and communicate with its own voice helps children develop better understanding about facial expressions.

WYSA by Touchkin (Wysa, https://www.wysa.io/) is an emotionally intelligent chatbot that uses AI and machine learning to provide personalised care for managing and improving user's mental health. Conversational chatbots can deliver psychological intervention tailored to a person's emotional state and clinical needs and help in providing support with behavioural illness, anxiety and depression.

California-based Cognoa's clinically validated machine learning app (Cognoa, https://cognoa.com/) helps identify autism among children as young as 18 months. It evaluates the child's behavioural health, analyses parent-provided information and videos of child's natural behaviour and provides an assessment of whether that child is developing at the right pace. It has even received categorization from the FDA as a diagnostic medical device for autism.

Virtual assistants like Siri, Cortana and Alexa have also proven to have the appropriate skill sets to communicate with ASD individuals however they were not primarily developed to cater to these people (Judith Newman, 2014). Table 3 includes a list of few robots and apps working in the field of autism, and their website respectively.

Limitations of AI for Treating Autism

Effectiveness of AI for treating autism largely depends on its outcomes. Although, AI based tools have the potential to support autistic children, they do have few shortcomings.

1. AI-based therapies are in development but are not yet available at a reasonable cost as they involve creating and training robots to interact and improve the ability of autistic children to identify facial expressions, interact socially, and respond appropriately to social cues.

Table 3. Some of the apps and robots in the field of autism

S No.	Robots	Website
1	Nao	https://www.softbankrobotics.com/emea/en/nao
2	Keepon	https://beatbots.net/my-keepon
3	Bandit	http://robotics.usc.edu/interaction/robots/
4	Milo	https://www.robokind.com/robots4autism/meet-milo
5	QTrobot	https://luxai.com/qt-robot-for-autism/
	Apps	**Website**
1	Cognoa	https://cognoa.com/
2	WYSA	https://www.wysa.io/
3	Proloquo2Go	https://www.assistiveware.com/products/proloquo2go
4	ABC Autismo	https://play.google.com/store/apps/details?id=com.dokye.abcautismo&hl=en&gl=US
5	Prism	https://www.etc.cmu.edu/projects/prism/

2. As the field of AI is constantly progressing, its use has rapidly spread in the healthcare sector, for example early cancer detection. However, there's lack of sufficiently large data to train the machine-learning models to predict ASD.
3. AI-based apps are available for any smart phone user but
   a. the amount of screen time needs to be taken care of,
   b. the children must be able enough to read, understand and have the will to follow the instructions given in the app which requires a certain level of understanding that might not be present in many children with autism.
4. While studies have shown high accuracy in identifying individuals with and without ASD, challenges regarding its feasibility in the market and among people needs to be resolved before fully integrating AI methods into the healthcare systems.

SCOPE FOR FUTURE RESEARCH AND DEVELOPMENT

- Advanced versions of voice-command technology like Google Assistant, Cortona can be incorporated into the discussed hands-free cursor utility, programmed accordingly to increase convenience in opening or closing tabs or websites, passing voice commands to play/pause the video etc. This might not be that helpful for the people with ASD who find it difficult to communicate through speech but can be beneficial for some autistic people who don't face such difficulties and also for other people with motor disabilities.

    - MIT researchers have developed a machine-learning application and a computer interface which performs real-time speech-to-text conversion without verbal communication using a face-mounted device (Larry Hardesty, 2018).
- Research is being conducted on using BCI for helping ASD patients and results include successful engagement and consistency in tasks (Oscar Schwartz, The Guardian(2019), Amaral C et al. 2018). A Brain Computer Interface, in layman terms can be understood as mind-reading technology, is a device that translates brain signals into commands for the application and allows for direct communication between the brain and a machine. It can be used to achieve improvements in identification of social clues and overall social behaviour. For example, using social games together with a BCI setup. An EEG (electroencephalographic) BCI can be used to (Amaral C et al. 2018):
    - Train social cognition skills
    - Decrease ATEC (Autism Treatment Evaluation Checklist) and symptoms which include sociability, sensory/cognitive awareness, physical health &behaviour.
    - Improve Adapted Behaviour Composite scores
    - Decrease depression (from POMS; Profile Of Mood States) and mood disturbance (BDI; Beck Depression Inventory)
- AI can help autistic people communicate their thoughts without actually speaking. This can be integrated into typical therapy sessions to help the therapists analyse the patient even better during or after their interaction. Researchers at Carnegie Mellon University have worked on reading complex thoughts based on brain activation patterns and output text accordingly. The study showed that complex thinking could enable its AI to predict the next sentence in the thought process (Wang, J. et al. 2017).
- Behaviour Imaging, an Idaho company, uses Naturalistic Observation Diagnostic Assessment (NODA) which is a tool in a smartphone application which allows parents to upload videos of their children for observation (Behavior Imaging Solutions: NODA, https://www.nodaautismdiagnosis.com/). They've developed AI algorithms to examine child's behaviour and point out specific behaviours to the clinicians that might otherwise have been missed.
- Thoughtful games may be created that require controlled gestures or body movements to play, which may help in reducing repetitive and impulsive actions. Reward-based games may be created to incorporate discipline, attention and patience.

- Advanced and more studies regarding aspects of brain function and development that are altered in people with ASD need to be conducted to understand and cater the autistic lives better and also develop technologies accordingly.

CONCLUSION

Manifold Artificial Intelligence advancements have been developed to help autistic children with their diagnosis, treatment and growth. Despite ongoing medical researches, no drugs have been identified yet to specifically treat autism, so, parents majorly rely on personal therapy and counselling as solutions.

AI-based interventions have helped autistic children, therapists and the parents by

1. Providing better assessment results and reports of the child.
2. Providing treatment strategies and suggestions, early.
3. The company of humanoid robots and virtual assistants to stay occupied with, get educated, and improve on the deficit skills along with the sense of a controlled environment.

AI can help healthcare professionals understand ASD better and support in executing advanced screening, diagnosis and treatment process. But before incorporating them into standard research and clinical settings, there exists a need to develop economically feasible AI-based interventions which could be exercised by maximum people.

The hands-free utility introduced is already being used by many people including people dealing with Amputations, Arthritis, Spinal Cord Injuries, Sclerosis and more. The chapter aims to raise awareness for the inclusion of such hands-free utilities for the autistic people as well. It is also to bring it to the concern of Computer Science engineers and researchers to work and contribute in developing the discussed resources explicitly for the people dealing with ASD. The proposed basic model of the "Mouse-less Cursor Control using Facial Movements" has certain limitations to be worked upon before being incorporated into systems for a wide user base.

Animouse, Smyle Mouse and other discussed innovations, which are already helping people with disabilities, are immaculate examples to understand the working of the discussed "Mouse-less Cursor Control" utility and evaluate its benefits for autistic children. Many autistic children who have speech-impairment and also cannot type or operate the computer using its mouse can leverage the hands-free mouse utility. They can take assistance from Human Computer Interaction and Brain Computer Interface technologies to express themselves, by transcribing their thoughts and emotions and assist other people understand them, perform tasks like web-surfing, creating virtual art & graphics and indulge in other activities available using computer and internet. Above all, be able to acquire employment and even create opportunities for others like them.

Development in the field of Brain Computer Interface can greatly benefit the society as a whole but especially the differently-abled and elder people. It can help tackle the gap between normal people and those who struggle with neuromuscular impairments, poor communication due to speech impairment, inability to write/type or similar challenges, by its potential to convert complex thoughts into texts or understandable literature.

More studies and researches are required to be conducted in the field of autism as insufficient significant data is available to train the AI-algorithms. "Mouse-less Cursor" technology (an application of Human Computer Interaction) and the field of "Brain Computer Interface" should also be included under the ongoing research topics in order to explore their advantages and benefits for the autistic children. Cumulative efforts from researchers of different fields including Autism, Psychology (Healthcare), and Computer Science are expected to develop more AI-assisted intervention technologies.

REFERENCES

ABC News. (2012, Aug). *Non-verbal girl with Autism speaks through her computer.* https://www.youtube.com/watch?v=xMBzJleeOno

Abrams, M., & Saunders, Z. (2018). Teacher for Children with Autism. *Mechanical Engineering (New York, N.Y.), 140*(12), 35. doi:10.1115/1.2018-DEC-4

Akshay, L. C. (2018, Oct). *Mouse Cursor Control Using Facial Movements — An HCI Application.* https://towardsdatascience.com/mouse-control-facial-movements-hci-app-c16b0494a971

Amaral, C., Mouga, S., Simões, M., Pereira, H.C., Bernardino, I., Quental, H., Playle, R., McNamara, R., Oliveira, G., & Castelo-Branco, M. (2018, July). A Feasibility Clinical Trial to Improve Social Attention in Autistic Spectrum Disorder (ASD) Using a Brain Computer Interface. *Front Neurosci., 13*(12), 477. doi:10.3389/fnins.2018.00477

Aniket Eknath Kudale. (2015, Aug). *Animouse.* https://github.com/aniketkudale/Animouse

Asthana, A., Marks, T. K., Jones, M. J., Tieu, K. H., & Rohith, M. V. (2011, November). Fully automatic pose-invariant face recognition via 3D pose normalization. In *2011 International Conference on Computer Vision* (pp. 937-944). IEEE. 10.1109/ICCV.2011.6126336

Basak, S. (2017, Feb) Mouse control with gesture. *Ishara - Mouse Control with Gesture*. https://github.com/saikatbsk/Ishara#readme

Behavior Imaging Solutions. (n.d.). *The Remote Autism Assessment Platform: NODA*. https://www.nodaautismdiagnosis.com/

Bender, L., Goldschmidt, L., Sankar, D. V. S., & Freedman, A. M. (1962). Treatment of Autistic Schizophrenic Children with LSD-25 and UML-491. In J. Wortis (Ed.), *Recent Advances in Biological Psychiatry*. Springer. doi:10.1007/978-1-4684-8306-2_17

Berg, T., & Belhumeur, P. N. (2012, September). Tom-vs-Pete Classifiers and Identity-Preserving Alignment for Face Verification. In BMVC (Vol. 2, p. 7). doi:10.5244/C.26.129

Buescher, A. V., Cidav, Z., Knapp, M., & Mandell, D. S. (2014, August). Costs of autism spectrum disorders in the United Kingdom and the United States. *JAMA Pediatrics*, *168*(8), 721–728. doi:10.1001/jamapediatrics.2014.210 PMID:24911948

Cao, C., Hou, Q., & Zhou, K. (2014). Displaced dynamic expression regression for real-time facial tracking and animation. *ACM Transactions on Graphics*, *33*(4), 1–10. doi:10.1145/3450626.3459806

Cao, X., Wei, Y., Wen, F., & Sun, J. (2014). Face alignment by explicit shape regression. *International Journal of Computer Vision*, *107*(2), 177–190. doi:10.100711263-013-0667-3

CDC. (2020, Feb). *Screening and Diagnosis of Autism Spectrum Disorder for Healthcare Providers*. https://www.cdc.gov/ncbddd/autism/hcp-screening.html

Cognoa. (n.d.). https://cognoa.com/

Cootes, T. F., Edwards, G. J., & Taylor, C. J. (2001, June). Active appearance models. *IEEE Transactions on Pattern Analysis and Machine Intelligence*, *23*(6), 681–685. doi:10.1109/34.927467

Cootes, T. F., Taylor, C. J., Cooper, D. H., & Graham, J. (1995). Active shape models-their training and application. *Computer Vision and Image Understanding*, *61*(1), 38–59. doi:10.1006/cviu.1995.1004

CREA Software Systems. (n.d.). *EVA Facial Mouse PRO*. https://play.google.com/store/apps/details?id=com.crea_si.eva_facial_mouse

Davenport, T., & Kalakota, R. (2019, June). The potential for artificial intelligence in healthcare. *Future Healthcare Journal*, *6*(2), 94–98. doi:10.7861/futurehosp.6-2-94 PMID:31363513

Dlib. (n.d.). *C ++ Library*. http://dlib.net/

Dollár, P., Welinder, P., & Perona, P. (2010, June). Cascaded pose regression. In *2010 IEEE Computer Society Conference on Computer Vision and Pattern Recognition* (pp. 1078-1085). IEEE.

Duquette, A., Michaud, F., & Mercier, H. (2008). Exploring the use of a mobile robot as an imitation agent with children with low-functioning autism. *Autonomous Robots*, *24*(2), 147–157. doi:10.100710514-007-9056-5

Eisenberg, L. (1957). The fathers of autistic children. *The American Journal of Orthopsychiatry*, *27*(4), 715–724. doi:10.1111/j.1939-0025.1957.tb05539.x PMID:13470021

Fakoor, R., Ladhak, F., Nazi, A., & Huber, M. (2013). Using deep learning to enhance cancer diagnosis and classification. *Proceedings of the ICML Workshop on the Role of Machine Learning in Transforming Healthcare*.

Falconer, J. (2013, May). *Nao Robot Goes to School to Help Kids With Autism*. https://spectrum.ieee.org/automaton/robotics/humanoids/aldebaran-robotics-nao-robot-autism-solution-for-kids

Fernández, A., Usamentiaga, R., Carús, J. L., & Casado, R. (2016). Driver distraction using visual-based sensors and algorithms. *Sensors (Basel)*, *16*(11), 1805. doi:10.339016111805 PMID:27801822

Fernández, A., Usamentiaga, R., Carús, J. L., & Casado, R. (2016). Driver distraction using visual-based sensors and algorithms. *Sensors (Basel)*, *16*(11), 1805. doi:10.339016111805 PMID:27801822

Hanson, D., Mazzei, D., Garver, C., Ahluwalia, A., De Rossi, D., Stevenson, M., & Reynolds, K. (2012, June). Realistic humanlike robots for treatment of ASD, social training, and research; shown to appeal to youths with ASD, cause physiological arousal, and increase human-to-human social engagement. *Proceedings of the 5th ACM international conference on pervasive technologies related to assistive environments (PETRA'12)*.

Hardesty, L. (2018, Apr). *Computer system transcribes words users "speak silently"*. https://news.mit.edu/2018/computer-system-transcribes-words-users-speak-silently-0404#:~:text=MIT%20researchers%20have%20developed%20a,does%20not%20actually%20speak%20aloud.&text=The%20signals%20are%20fed%20to,particular%20signals%20with%20particular%20words

Hockey, G. R. J., Hockey, R., Gaillard, A. W., & Burov, O. (Eds.). (2003). *Operator functional state: the assessment and prediction of human performance degradation in complex tasks* (Vol. 355). IOS Press.

Hu, Y., Jiang, D., Yan, S., & Zhang, L. (2004, May). Automatic 3D reconstruction for face recognition. In *Sixth IEEE International Conference on Automatic Face and Gesture Recognition, 2004. Proceedings.* (pp. 843-848). IEEE.

Huang, G. B., & Learned-Miller, E. (2014). *Labeled faces in the wild: Updates and new reporting procedures.* Dept. Comput. Sci., Univ. Massachusetts Amherst, *Tech. Rep*, *14*(003).

Instruments, O. (n.d.). *HeadMouse® Nano Wireless Head Controlled Access Works on Computers, Smartphones, Tablets – Everything!* https://www.orin.com/access/headmouse/#:~:text=HeadMouse%20replaces%20the%20standard%20computer,the%20mouse%20pointer%20follows%20along

Kamath & Dalwai. (2017, May). IAP Chapter of Neuro Developmental Pediatrics. *National Guidelines Autism.*

Kaur, K., & Pany, S. (2017). Computer-based intervention for autism spectrum disorder children and their social skills: A meta-analysis. *Scholarly Research Journal for Humanity Science & English Language.*, *4*(23). Advance online publication. doi:10.21922rjhsel.v4i23.9649

Kaur, R., & Kautish, S. (2019). Multimodal sentiment analysis: A survey and comparison. *International Journal of Service Science, Management, Engineering, and Technology*, *10*(2), 38–58. doi:10.4018/IJSSMET.2019040103

Kazemi, V., & Sullivan, J. (2014). One millisecond face alignment with an ensemble of regression trees. *2014 IEEE Conference on Computer Vision and Pattern Recognition*, 1867-1874. 10.1109/CVPR.2014.241

Kozima, H., Michalowski, M. P., & Nakagawa, C. (2009). Keepon. *International Journal of Social Robotics*, *1*(1), 3–18. doi:10.100712369-008-0009-8

Lefkovits, S., Lefkovits, L., & Emerich, S. (2017, April). Detecting the eye and its openness with Gabor filters. In *2017 5th International Symposium on Digital Forensic and Security (ISDFS)* (pp. 1-5). IEEE. 10.1109/ISDFS.2017.7916506

List of Files. (n.d.). http://dlib.net/files

Matsuda, S., Minagawa, Y., & Yamamoto, J. (2015). Gaze Behavior of Children with ASD toward Pictures of Facial Expressions. Autism Research and Treatment. doi:10.1155/2015/617190

Mihajlović, S., Kupusinac, A., Ivetić, D., & Berković, I. (2020). *The Use of Python in the field of Artificial Intelligence*. Academic Press.

Moreno, C. (2018). Use of HCI for the development of emotional skills in the treatment of Autism Spectrum Disorder. *Systematic Reviews*, 1–6. doi:10.23919/CISTI.2018.8399209

Mouse, S. (n.d.). https://smylemouse.com/

National Autistic Society. (2020, Aug). *Employing autistic people – a guide for employers.* https://www.autism.org.uk/advice-and-guidance/topics/employment/employing-autistic-people/employers

Newman, J. (2014, Oct). *To Siri, With Love*. https://www.nytimes.com/2014/10/19/fashion/how-apples-siri-became-one-autistic-boys-bff.html

Parsons. (2018, July). *The costs of autism strap many families.* Orlando Sentinels. https://www.orlandosentinel.com/health/get-healthy-orlando/os-families-cost-of-autism-20180702-story.html

Ramdoss, S., Lang, R., Mulloy, A., Franco, J., O'Reilly, M., Didden, R., & Lancioni, G. (2011). Use of Computer-Based Interventions to Teach Communication Skills to Children with Autism Spectrum Disorders: A Systematic Review. *Journal of Behavioral Education*, *20*(1), 55–76. doi:10.100710864-010-9112-7

Rani, S., & Kautish, S. (2018). Application of data mining techniques for prediction of diabetes-A review. *International Journal of Scientific Research in Computer Science, Engineering and Information Technology*, *3*(3), 1996–2004.

Rani, S., & Kautish, S. (2018, June). Association clustering and time series based data mining in continuous data for diabetes prediction. In *2018 second international conference on intelligent computing and control systems (ICICCS)* (pp. 1209-1214). IEEE. 10.1109/ICCONS.2018.8662909

Ren, S., Cao, X., Wei, Y., & Sun, J. (2016). Face alignment via regressing local binary features. *IEEE Transactions on Image Processing*, *25*(3), 1233–1245. doi:10.1109/TIP.2016.2518867 PMID:26800539

Reyana, A., & Kautish, S. (2021). *Corona virus-related Disease Pandemic: A Review on Machine Learning Approaches and Treatment Trials on Diagnosed Population for Future Clinical Decision Support*. Current Medical Imaging.

Reyana, A., Krishnaprasath, V. T., Kautish, S., Panigrahi, R., & Shaik, M. (2020). Decision-making on the existence of soft exudates in diabetic retinopathy. *International Journal of Computer Applications in Technology*, *64*(4), 375–381. doi:10.1504/IJCAT.2020.112684

Robokind. (n.d.). *A non-threatening way for learners with ASD to practice their communication and social skills*. https://www.robokind.com/robots4autism/meet-milo

Rosebrock. (2017a, Apr). *Eye blink detection with OpenCV, Python, and dlib*. Academic Press.

Rosebrock. (2017b, Apr). *Detect eyes, nose, lips, and jaw with dlib, OpenCV, and Python*. Academic Press.

Sagonas, C., Antonakos, E., Tzimiropoulos, G., Zafeiriou, S., & Pantic, M. (2016). 300 faces in-the-wild challenge: Database and results. *Image and Vision Computing*, *47*, 3–18. doi:10.1016/j.imavis.2016.01.002

Sagonas, C., Tzimiropoulos, G., Zafeiriou, S., & Pantic, M. (2013). A semi-automatic methodology for facial landmark annotation. In *Proceedings of the IEEE conference on computer vision and pattern recognition workshops* (pp. 896-903). 10.1109/CVPRW.2013.132

Sagonas, C., Tzimiropoulos, G., Zafeiriou, S., & Pantic, M. (2013). 300 faces in-the-wild challenge: The first facial landmark localization challenge. In *Proceedings of the IEEE International Conference on Computer Vision Workshops* (pp. 397-403). 10.1109/ICCVW.2013.59

Sampathkumar, A., Rastogi, R., Arukonda, S., Shankar, A., Kautish, S., & Sivaram, M. (2020). An efficient hybrid methodology for detection of cancer-causing gene using CSC for micro array data. *Journal of Ambient Intelligence and Humanized Computing*, *11*(11), 4743–4751. doi:10.100712652-020-01731-7

Schenkman, L. (2020, August). *Motor difficulties in autism, explained*. https://www.spectrumnews.org/news/motor-difficulties-in-autism-explained/

Schwartz, O. (2019, Oct). *Mind-reading tech? How private companies could gain access to our brains.* https://www.theguardian.com/technology/2019/oct/24/mind-reading-tech-private-companies-access-brains#:~:text=A%20BCI%20is%20a%20device,be%20recognized%20by%20the%20machine

Sharma, S. R., Gonda, X., & Tarazi, F. I. (2018, May). Autism Spectrum Disorder: Classification, diagnosis and therapy. *Pharmacology & Therapeutics*, *190*, 91–104. Advance online publication. doi:10.1016/j.pharmthera.2018.05.007 PMID:29763648

Sigafoos, J., Green, V. A., Edrisinha, C., & Lancioni, G. E. (2007). Flashback to the 1960s: LSD in the treatment of autism. *Developmental Neurorehabilitation*, *10*(1), 75–81. doi:10.1080/13638490601106277 PMID:17608329

Singh, A., Chandewar, C., & Pattarkine, P. (2018). Driver drowsiness alert system with effective feature extraction. *Int. JR in Emer. Sciences et Techniques (Paris)*, *5*(4), 26–31.

Sixty-Seventh World Health Assembly Geneva. (2014, May). *WHA67.8: Comprehensive and coordinated efforts for the management of autism spectrum disorders*. Palais des Nations.

Smith, V., & Sung, A. (2014). Computer Interventions for ASD. In V. Patel, V. Preedy, & C. Martin (Eds.), *Comprehensive Guide to Autism*. Springer., doi:10.1007/978-1-4614-4788-7_134

Soukupova, T., & Cech, J. (2016, February). *Eye blink detection using facial landmarks*. In 21st computer vision winter workshop, Rimske Toplice, Slovenia.

Tapus, A., Peca, A., Aly, A., Pop, C., Jisa, L., Pintea, S., ... David, D. O. (2012). Children with autism social engagement in interaction with Nao, an imitative robot: A series of single case experiments. *Interaction Studies: Social Behaviour and Communication in Biological and Artificial Systems*, *13*(3), 315–347. doi:10.1075/is.13.3.01tap

Viacam, E. (n.d.). https://eviacam.crea-si.com/index.php

Wainer, J., Robins, B., Amirabdollahian, F., & Dautenhahn, K. (2014, September). Using the Humanoid Robot KASPAR to Autonomously Play Triadic Games and Facilitate Collaborative Play Among Children With Autism. *IEEE Transactions on Autonomous Mental Development*, *6*(3), 183–199. doi:10.1109/TAMD.2014.2303116

Wang, J., Cherkassky, V. L., & Just, M. A. (2017). Predicting the brain activation pattern associated with the propositional content of a sentence: Modeling neural representations of events and states. *Human Brain Mapping*, *38*(10), 4865–4881. doi:10.1002/hbm.23692 PMID:28653794

Wysa. (n.d.). https://www.wysa.io/

Xiong, X., & De la Torre, F. (2013). Supervised descent method and its applications to face alignment. In *Proceedings of the IEEE conference on computer vision and pattern recognition* (pp. 532-539). 10.1109/CVPR.2013.75

Zhu, X., Lei, Z., Yan, J., Yi, D., & Li, S. Z. (2015). High-fidelity pose and expression normalization for face recognition in the wild. In *Proceedings of the IEEE conference on computer vision and pattern recognition* (pp. 787-796). IEEE.

Zhu, X., & Ramanan, D. (2012, June). *Face detection, pose estimation, and landmark localization in the wild. In 2012 IEEE conference on computer vision and pattern recognition*. IEEE.

KEY TERMS AND DEFINITIONS

Artificial Intelligence: Field within Computer Science that attempts to simulate and build enhanced human intelligence into machines.

Aspect Ratio: Ratio between the width and height of an image.

Autism Spectrum Disorder: Lifelong neurodevelopmental disorder characterised by repetitive patterns of behaviour and impaired development in communication, interaction, and understanding of social clues.

Brain-Computer Interface: A computer-based system used to translate brain signals into commands to an output device.

Facial Landmarks: Key points on face used to extract facial features.

Human-Computer Interaction: Technology field that studies the interaction between humans and computers and deals with the design, execution and assessment of computer systems.

Motor Difficulty: Inability to move and coordinate body movements in a normal manner.

Social Skills: Skills used to communicate and interact with each other including speech, gesture, body language, etc.

Chapter 9
Optimization of Machine Learning Models for Early Diagnosis of Autism Spectrum Disorder

Mohan Allam
https://orcid.org/0000-0002-3117-6047
Pondicherry University, India

M. Nandhini
Pondicherry University, India

M. Thangadarshini
Pondicherry Engineering College, India

ABSTRACT

Autism spectrum disorder is a syndrome related to interaction with people and repetitive behavior. ASD is diagnosed by health experts with the help of special practices that can be prolonged and costly. Researchers developed several ASD detection techniques by utilizing machine learning tools. ML provides the advanced algorithms that build automatic classification models. But disease prediction is a challenge for ML models due to the majority of the medical datasets including irrelevant features. Feature selection is a critical job in the predictive modeling for selecting a subset of significant features from the dataset. Recent feature selection techniques are using the optimization algorithms to improve the prediction rate of classification models. Most of the optimization algorithms make use of several controlling parameters that have to be tuned for improved productivity. In this chapter, a novel feature selection technique is proposed using binary teaching learning-based optimization algorithm that requires standard controlling parameters to acquire optimum features from ASD data.

DOI: 10.4018/978-1-7998-7460-7.ch009

INTRODUCTION

Autism Spectrum disorder (ASD) is a syndrome that is related to human neural structure developmental. A person with ASD normally faces several challenges connected to behavioral, communication and social constipation (Fadi, 2018). This problem has been growing rapidly among all ages of individuals. Most of the researchers are considering the hereditary and ecological traits may be the reasons for this disease. There are some other possibilities which leads the ASD are low weight at birth and aged parents. However, the exact origin of ASD has not been identified by experts. Autism can be diagnosed at any period of human lifetime. As said by experts, ASD distress starts with in the first two years of birth and persists to teens as well as middle age (Allison, 2012). The symptoms of this dilemma appear at the age of 3 years and will be able to remain for the long time. It would not be possible to successfully cure the patient having this disorder, though its impacts can be lowered for quite a while if the signs and symptoms are early diagnosed. Early diagnosis and therapy are the most significant measures to be adopted to decrease the impact of ASD disorder. There is absolutely no method of medical examination for the discovery of autism and evidences are typically identified through observation. In kids and teenagers, the signs of ASD are normally recognized by parents and educators in schools or colleges. The parents will consult the physicians regarding the issue and follow the precautions given by specialists.

The procedure of diagnosing people with autism is sluggish, involving clinical resources and analysis techniques. Therefore, it is assumed that a lot more individuals who are on the continuum stay unnoticed (Reyana & Kautish, 2021). There is an immediate requirement for sophisticated intelligent techniques that can provide the automatic diagnosis of ASD. These intelligent techniques can be used by doctors, educators, health care professionals, and relatives to comprehend the outcome of the diagnosis. The ASD diagnostic methods involve projecting statistics of people that are experiencing difficulties with ASD. These diagnostic tools (Sampathkumar et al 2020) will apply predetermined attributes comprising a class and a historical dataset. Moreover, the ASD diagnosis issue can be interpreted as a classification job in supervised learning. In this connection, the health practitioner will employ labelled instances of people as ASD victim or healthy to build a classifier by means of a ML system. The model is subsequently utilized to automatically predict the category of an unknown individual as accurately as possible.

The Machine Learning techniques are concerning in every real-time potential problem (Rani & Kautish, 2018), especially in the health sector. Furthermore, numerous machine learning models have been developed for diagnosing a variety of diseases like lung cancer, breast cancer, Alzheimer's disease and Melanoma (Mohan,

2017). The productivity of a machine learning model particularly differs with the attributes or features engaged in the training procedure. All the features of the data might not be linked to the specified problem. These machine learning prototypes are challenging by the needless information in the data produced from different sources. Additionally, the overall performance of the computer-assisted disease diagnostic tool decreases with high-dimensional data. Feature selection models will manage these huge data challenges by separating the unrelated attributes from the data. Numerous feature selection approaches have been suggested in the literature to discover optimal features from the datasets. Among the widespread feature selection techniques, the evolutionary algorithm-centered practices outperformed with well-known classification algorithms.

The most common evolutionary algorithm namely, GA is used by many investigators for choosing better features from different medical data. The GA will strengthen the process of exploring the informative features or predictors in the attribute space. Generally, optimization procedures make use of a variety of computational parameters that are specific to the algorithm in combination with the usual controlling parameters throughout the operation. These parameters perform a vital function during the course of feature selection and impact on the operation of ML models. The BTLBO is a metaheuristic algorithm that is straightforward and requires just the prevalent parameters like the number of solutions within the population and halting conditions. The idea of BTLBO has proved to be adopted to shorten the requirement of setting up the parameter's values through the feature selection procedure. The suggested model explores through the feature (solution) space for choosing optimal features.

In this chapter, several ML models based on Support Vector Machines (SVM), Naïve Bayes (NB), k-Nearest Neighbours (KNN) and Decision Trees (DT) algorithms are developed and enhanced with optimized feature selection models for prompt diagnosis of ASD. The feature selection models use well-known evolutionary and metaheuristic optimization algorithms like GA and BTLBO. The key objective of the proposed feature selection models is to choose an optimal subgroup of predictors or attributes from the solution (feature) space. The continued sections will explain the recommended work of building optimized machine learning models using optimal feature selection. Section 2 discusses the earlier research on automatic ASD diagnosis with the machine learning models and feature selection for classification models using different evolutionary algorithms. Section 3 addresses the proposed machine learning models with respect to GA and BTLBO based feature selection methods. The experimental setup and discussion of results on various ASD datasets are specified in section 4. The final section gives the summary and the future scope of other evolutionary algorithms for feature selection to build machine learning models.

BACKGROUND

The researchers of emotional, consciousness, and the scientific disciplines have established several testing methodologies to identify the possible autistic traits in the individuals (Baron, 2001). The STAT – "Screening Tool for Autism in Toddlers & Young Children" is an analytically developed, collaborative measure which has been established to diagnose for autism in children aged between 24 –36 month period. It is designed to be used by social service workers that operate with adolescent in the evaluation environments. There have been a handful surveys taking into account of the machine learning for ASD screening in the last few years. Suman and Sarfaraz (2020) developed several machine learning models for diagnosing and evaluation of autism disorder in various age groups of individuals. They have assessed the classification models using various performance metrics such as specificity, sensitivity and accuracy. Mythili et al. (2015) have experimented on ASD problem using various classification algorithms of WEKA tool. They have identified multiple levels of autism in the analysis of students. Ugur and Dang (2019) implemented several classification models for early detection of ASD and tested on 3 datasets of the UCI database. Jayalakshmi et al. (2019) discussed about the problems of autism in human life and implemented several predictive models. The authors evaluated the performance of models using different classification measures. Mohamed et al. (2021) performed feature selection and applied machine learning on home videos for diagnosing autism remotely. Nadire et al. (2021) reviewed the latest articles on the implementation of machine learning in the behavioral evaluation of ASD, and emphasized widespread challenges in the findings, and suggested essential factors for real-life applications of machine learning based ASD diagnostic techniques.

Genetic algorithm has evidenced a considerable improvement across a range of local search methods (Kenneth, 1988). The adaptive search ability of GA exploits the initial unknown feature space into promising feature subspaces. The GA is fundamentally a domain neutral search method, that is perfect for applications in which the domain understanding is challenging or unfeasible to provide. Cheng-Lung and Chieh-Jen (2006) performed feature selection and parameters optimization concurrently on various real-world datasets using GA. The authors compared the results of GA with grid algorithm. GA-based features considerably increased the classification accuracy of SVM. Adriano et al. (2010) examined the usage of GA for optimal feature subset selection and parameter optimization of machine learning models. The authors achieved higher classification accuracies for the effort estimates of software projects using various benchmark datasets. The GA based feature selection enhanced the performance of the machine learning algorithms and significantly decreased the number of original features for all the data.

Several investigators (Reyana et al, 2020) also applied TLBO algorithm for choosing useful features from the data in different domains. Shouheng et al. (2017) established a hybrid feature selection method employing harmony search and TLBO to handle high dimensional data. Ender and Tansel (2019) introduced a novel hybrid algorithm with an integration of TLBO and extreme learning machines in order to classify various category problems of UCI data. A new multi-objective feature selection method was built by employing TLBO for binary classification applications (Hakan, 2018). This technique accomplished improved outcomes in comparison with previous algorithms such as the GA & Tabu search. Suresh et al. (2013) recommended a feature selection technique by combining the TLBO & rough set theory. Mohan and Nandhini (2020) improved the BTLBO by integrating multiple teachers for selecting better features from the data. Saeid et al. (2012) implemented an intrusion detection system that utilizes the NCA for feature transformation and genetic algorithm for feature selection. This technique attained improved outcomes compare to existing practices. Mohan and Nandhini (2018) performed feature optimization using TLBO algorithm for diagnosis of cancerous tumors in the patients. Mohan and Nandhini (2018) implemented an optimal feature selection model built on binary teaching learning based optimization algorithm.

The majority of study reviewed previously employed traditional machine learning methodologies and therefore are restricted in their efficiency and effectiveness. It is clear from the reviewed section that there is certainly a necessity to optimize the potential of machine learning models for the diagnosis of ASD in the world's population. In this effort, efficiency of multiple ML models has been contrasted with various ASD datasets available in the UCI repository. Finally, the effectiveness of the ML models that are optimized with the evolutionary feature selection methods are evaluated by way of classification measures. This chapter is mainly concentrated on optimizing the performance of machine learning models by selecting significant features from data using BTLBO algorithm for ASD diagnosis.

MACHINE LEARNING BASED ASD DIAGNOSIS

Machine Learning (ML) is an emerging area of artificial intelligence (AI) which facilitates computers in developing models from the past data to automate the decision-making activity. Computer-assisted systems with AI has played important role for early detection of diseases in the medical sector.

Machine Learning Without Feature Selection

A simple ML model with various classification algorithms for ASD diagnosis is presented in the Figure 1. These models learn and enhance their performance

Figure 1. A simple Machine Learning model without feature selection for ASD diagnosis

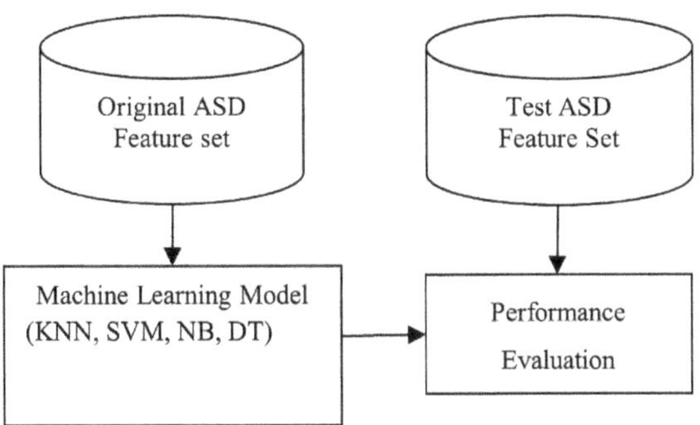

utilizing numerous features available in the data. The performance of ML algorithms is evaluated by using test datasets.

Machine Learning With Evolutionary Based Feature Selection

Feature Selection methods look for the whole feature space and finds the probable attributes that are appropriate for the application. These specified beneficial features are drawn from the original data which includes complete features to build a best dataset (Kaur & Kautish, 2019). The whole process of choosing the appropriate features from the solution space will occur in multiple generations. The fitness of individuals is calculated based on the type of feature selection methods such as classification accuracies or errors in wrapper techniques and weights of the features in filter methods in each single generation. Individuals obtaining higher fitness values will be taken to the following generation with the suitable informative attributes. The subsequent generations will hold the finest individuals with the best possible attributes. An evolutionary algorithm is expected to optimize feature selection

Figure 2. A Machine Learning model with feature selection for ASD diagnosis

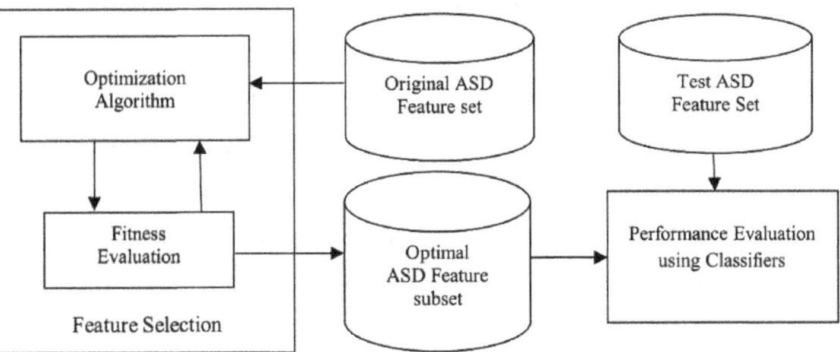

process and build a powerful decision-making system. A ML model with feature selection support for auto diagnosis of ASD in humans is illustrated in Figure 2.

Feature Selection Based on GA

GA is a known meta-heuristic algorithm motivated by the fact of survival of the fittest. GA is associated with the category of an evolutionary algorithm. The key activities in GA comprise, chromosome encoding, establishing a population, fitness estimation, choosing the solutions from the population and doing genetic operations such as crossover and mutation. The flow of GA is as indicated below.

Genetic Algorithm

1. Start
2. Assign preliminary solutions to the population
3. Assess fitness cost for all solutions in the population as per,

$$Fitness\left(Solution\right) = Classification\,Error\left(Solution\right)$$

4. Go again until the criteria specified are attained
5. Choose solutions from the population
6. Crossover the attributes of solutions to constitute offspring
7. Mutate the solutions to constitute offspring
8. Decide the best solutions for the future generation
9. Finish

The population consist of randomly produced initial solutions described as chromosomes. The solutions are encoded through the use of binary strings that contain 1's and 0's representing the participation and nonparticipation of a specific feature from the data relates to that position. The selection operator is designed to choose good solutions to be maintained and permitted to reproduce in the population for the next generations. The weak solutions will be removed in the population at the same time holding the population size fixed. Most commonly employed selection methods are roulette wheel, rank and tournament selection operators. The crossover operation explains the switch of specific bits (genes) between the two strings in a certain way to generate two children. Crossover works by means of indiscriminately selecting a point from two selected parent strings and swapping the left-over segments of the parent strings to generate new offspring. Thus, crossover promotes the features of two parent solutions to generate two similar offspring. The mutation operation is the occasional infusion of additional features into the solution sequences to conserve diversity throughout the population. The mutation operator turns the bit value at a certain spot in the solution string with the inverse bit to generate a new solution. The mutation operator is skilled to preserve the variety of the population as well as improving the probability of achieving global optimization. Mutation operates by indiscriminately changing one or several bits of a chosen solution. It works as a population distress operator and is requires for integrating the additional information into the population. This operator prevents any rigidity that could happen during the search activity. The primary objective of the established model involves lowering the number of attributes for training and testing the classification model as well as enhance the effectiveness of the classification model with a subset of attributes.

The machine learning model with GA based feature selection for early detection of autism in people is shown in Figure 3. The complete feature set includes ASD diagnosis attributes of all individuals in the dataset. Initial population is generated with a specific number of binary strings representing the availability of features in the ASD data. Further, the fitness of each solution string in the population is evaluated. The proposed model uses various classification algorithms for fitness assessment. Different operations of GA are conducted to discover new solutions in the population. These operations will be performed for a determined number of times referred to as generations. In every generation, solutions with the maximum fitness cost will be disseminated towards the future population. The algorithm concludes with an optimal solution representing ideal features.

Figure 3. A Machine Learning model with GA based feature selection for ASD diagnosis

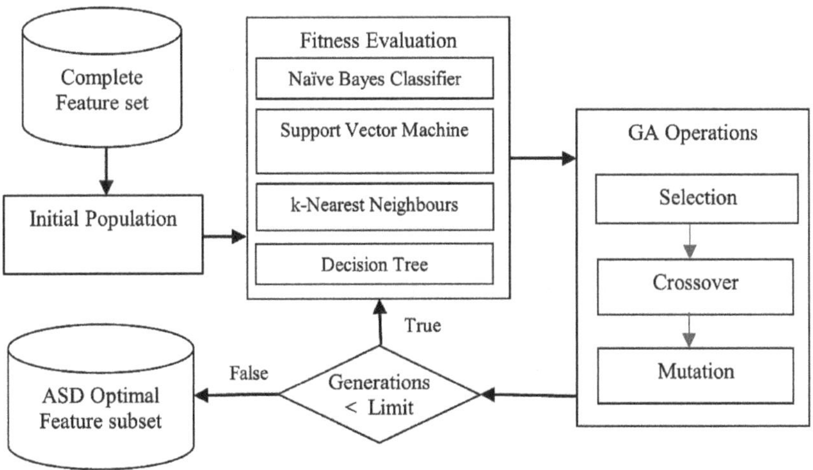

Feature Selection Based on BTLBO

The TLBO is a population reinforced optimization algorithm that hardly depends on any local factors. A binary interpretation of TLBO algorithm has been used to examine the feature space for choosing the important subgroup of attributes. The procedure operates in two stages, referred to as a teacher and learner stages, for those wishing to explore the whole data. The algorithm finishes with a specific number of repetitions by choosing an individual with informative attributes. Every individual has 'n' number of predictors (features (f):1 to n) and 'e' examples (individuals (i) from 1 to e). The variable 'u' restricts the process in accordance with the repetitions. The functioning steps (S1, S2, ..., S6) of BTLBO algorithm is demonstrated as follows,

S1: Assign the initial binary individuals by indicating attributes as $X_{f,i}$ in the population & End condition.

S2: For each repetition u, estimate the mean for features independently by $M_{f,u}$.

S3: Assess the fitness of individuals with the Equation 1.

$$Fitness\left(X_{f,i,u}\right) = Error\left(X_{f,i,u}\right) \tag{1}$$

Teacher Phase:

S4: Fit all solutions (Students) concerning the top individual (or Teacher)

1. Prefer the best student (high fitness) from the class as a teacher.
2. Infer the mean difference for complete features utilizing the leading student as demonstrated in the Equation 2.

$$Dif\_Mn_{f,i,u} = r_v\left(X_{f,itop,u} - T_F M_{f,u}\right) \tag{2}$$

Here, $X_{f,itop,u}$ is the best individual in the field f. TF defines the teaching factor and r_u specifies the random number.

3. The top individual serves as a teacher to instructs the leftover learners using Equation (3).

$$\begin{aligned} X'_{f,i,u} &= 0\, when\, X_{f,i,u} + Dif\_Mn_{f,u} < 0.5 \\ X'_{f,i,u} &= 1\, when\, X_{f,i,u} + Dif\_Mn_{f,u} \geq 0.5 \end{aligned} \tag{3}$$

Here, $X'_{f,i,u}$ is the modified value of $X_{f,i,u}$

4. If $X'_{f,i,u}$ is beneficial than $X_{f,i,u}$, employ the revised value otherwise, remain the last value.

Learner Phase:

S5: Update each individual utilizing fellow learners in the class by Equations (4) and (5).

1. Nominate 2 entities G and H with a prerequisite for $X'_{tot-G,k} \neq X'_{tot-H,u}$ randomly.

Here, $X'_{tot-G,u}$, $X'_{tot-H,u}$ are renewed quantities of $X_{tot-G,u}$, $X_{tot-H,u}$ for G and H correspondingly.

2. If $X'_{tot-G,v}$ outperforms than $X'_{tot-H,u}$

$$X''_{f,G,u} = 0 \; when \; X'_{f,G,u} + r_u \left(X'_{f,G,u} - X'_{f,H,u} \right) < 0.5$$

$$X''_{f,G,u} = 1 \; when \; X'_{f,G,u} + r_u \left(X'_{f,G,u} - X'_{f,H,u} \right) \geq 0.5 \qquad (4)$$

otherwise,

$$X''_{f,G,u} = 0 \; when \; X'_{f,G,u} + r_u \left(X'_{f,H,u} - X'_{f,G,u} \right) < 0.5$$

$$X''_{f,G,u} = 1 \; when \; X'_{f,G,u} + r_u \left(X'_{f,H,u} - X'_{f,G,u} \right) \geq 0.5 \qquad (5)$$

3. If $X''_{f,G,v}$ is more beneficial than $X'_{f,G,v}$ employ the revised value otherwise, retain the last value.

S6: If the ending conditions fulfilled, present the conclusion otherwise, move on to S2

In BTLBO, the population is in the binary level that presents the involvement of a particular attribute in the individual. Every solution in the population includes binary bit structures that are exactly the same number of features in the data.

The binary bits (1, 2) imply the occurrence and lack of a certain feature of the individual. In the early stage, solutions will be trained by the best performer in terms of difference mean. If the imparted difference is greater than a threshold point (0.5), the solution will pursue the instructor solution in accordance with the conditions of the features that are available as demonstrated in the Equation (3). In the subsequent stage, the learners will evolve and refresh the content with the twin communication as demonstrated in the Equations (4) and (5). The BTLBO focuses primarily on 'discovery as well as exploitation' of the feature combination for choosing the right mix of subgroup of features by mimicking the standard the educational method of a learner from educators and peers in education. The best pertinent features in solutions will instruct the leftover solutions to establish a minimized feature subset. The suggested feature selection technique utilizing BTLBO algorithms is illustrated in Figure 4.

The feature selection by using the BTLBO algorithm begins with the initial configuration of the population, defining the appropriate number of individuals, repetitions and the value of teaching factor. The total of 1's in the solution sequence reveals the features chosen in the solution. The BTLBO algorithm is structured into two sections mentioned as teacher & learner phases. In the opening phase, competence is assessed for all individuals in the solution region by the assistance of the classification algorithm. The solution that has the highest fitness cost will

Figure 4. Machine Learning model with BTLBO based feature selection

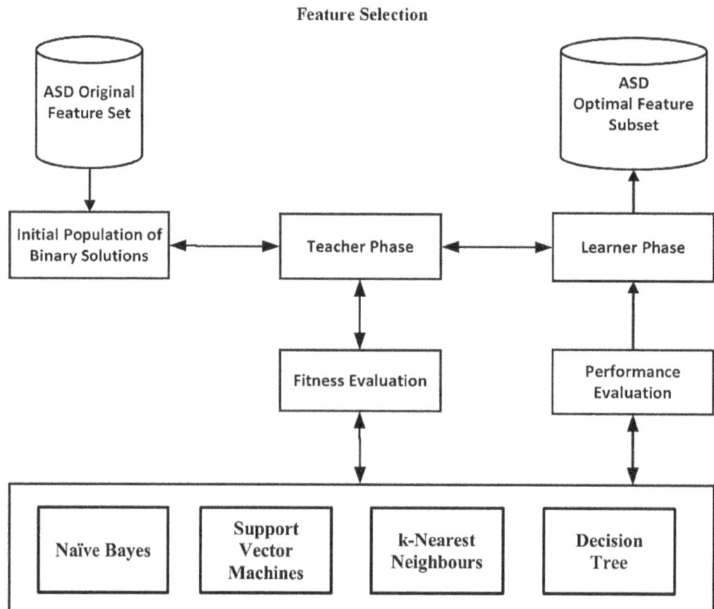

be determined as a tutor. The tutor will estimate the difference mean (Equation 2) for all features of the solutions in the population and revise the leftover individuals with respect to the mathematical operation shown in Equation (3). The revised solution will be compared to the older one to retain the most beneficial in the survive population of the present generation.

In the learner phase, all solutions are revised with a randomly-chosen solutions utilizing Equation (4) and Equation (5) in connection to the fitness evaluated by the classifiers. Now, relate the preliminary and revised fitness scores of solutions to nominate into the population for the following generation. Finally, verify the termination condition (generation count) at the conclusion on each iteration and wrap up the algorithm procedure by choosing the best solution with an optimum subset of features containing the highest fitness values. The features with the better fitness will have greater efficiency in managing the machine learning models. To demonstrate above-mentioned accomplishments, various experiments have been carried out utilizing the ASD datasets for diagnosing autism early in the stages. The findings are compared without having to use any feature selection method against different optimization algorithms and exhibited in the manner of tables as well as graphs in the following section.

EXPERIMENTAL ANALYSIS

The performance of ML models with respect to GA and BTLBO based feature selection are evaluated by employing a variety of performing measures such as accuracy, recall, precision, F-Measure and AUC (Area under the curve) values on 3 ASD datasets of UCI data . The efficiency of ML models with and without feature selection also compared at the end.

Datasets and Description

In this research, the ASD datasets of well-known UCI machine learning archive (Thabtah, 2017)has been utilized to scrutinize the performance of the suggested diagnosis system. The child dataset is formed by 292 examples, adolescent dataset is formed by 104 examples and adult dataset is formed by 704 examples for the classification of autism using the features chosen by BTLBO algorithm. The effectiveness of the feature selection techniques is analyzed with the results derived from the ML models developed by utilizing NB, SVM, KNN and DT algorithms. The names of the attribute and the explanation are stipulated in Table 1.

Table 1. ASD Features Specification

Features	Details
F1: Age	Age of individual (years)
F2: Gender	Gender of individual (Male / Female)
F3: Ethnicity	Record of familiar ethnicities
F4: Born with Jaundice	Candidate born along with jaundice (True / False)
F5: Family member with PDD	If some close family member experiences a PDD (True / False)
F6: Who is completing the test	Family, Candidate, Care provider, health care professionals
F7: Country of residence	Record of geographic regions
F8: Used the screening app earlier	If the candidate has utilized a testing application (True / False)
F9: Screening Method Type	The kind of testing techniques preferred depending on age group (0-infant, 12-child, 2-adolescent, 3-adult)
F10: Ans (Q1)	The response to the question made on the testing technique applied
F11: Ans (Q2)	The response to the question made on the testing technique applied
F12: Ans (Q3)	The response to the question made on the testing technique applied
F13: Ans (Q4)	The response to the question made on the testing technique applied
F14: Ans (Q5)	The response to the question made on the testing technique applied
F15: Ans (Q6)	The response to the question made on the testing technique applied
F16: Ans (Q7)	The response to the question made on the testing technique applied
F17: Ans (Q8)	The response to the question made on the testing technique applied
F18: Ans (Q9)	The response to the question made on the testing technique applied
F19: Ans (Q10)	The response to the question made on the testing technique applied
F20: Screening Score	The end score attained based on the assessing algorithm of the testing technique employed.

Evaluation of Machine Learning Models Without Feature Selection

Several machine learning models are developed using KNN, NB, SVM as well as DT classifiers and trained with all autism features of the children, adolescent and adults available in the UCI data. These ML models have been evaluated by computing various classification measures with test data. The accuracy of a classification algorithm could be evaluated as the proportion of the true estimates to the overall estimates produced on the test data. Precision is the proportion of real accurate projections against the complete positive identifications. Recall is the properly categorized against real positives in the test data. F-Measure will be calculated utilizing recall &

precision as a weighted harmonic mean. The Receiver Operating Characteristic (ROC) curve estimates the efficiency of a classifier on the objective of two components, referred to as the true positive rate (TPR) and false positive rate (FPR). The AUC evaluates the region under the ROC curve and the values varies from 0 (suggesting 100% false predictions) to 1 (suggesting 100% accurate estimates).

Assessment of ML Models on ASD Screening Data of Children

Various classification measures attained by the models on autism data of children without employing any feature selection technique are depicted in Table 2. The NB model performed best with an accuracy of 94.25% and also accomplished better values for remaining metrics than the other models. The AUC scores are almost comparable and greater than 0.9 for all the implemented ML models.

Table 2. Performance measures of ML models with children autism data

Performance Measures	Machine Learning Models			
	KNN	**NB**	**SVM**	**DT**
Accuracy (%)	79.31	**94.25**	86.2	93.1
Precision	0.85	0.983	0.921	0.903
Recall	0.739	0.891	0.795	0.979
F-Measure	0.79	0.942	0.853	0.94
AUC	0.912	0.993	0.973	0.969

Assessment of ML Models on ASD Screening Data of Adolescent

The classification measures attained by the models on autism data of adolescent with all the features in the dataset are specified in Table 3. The decision tree model achieved better accuracy with a value of 90.32%. It also achieved comparable results with precision, F-Measure and AUC values. The recall and AUC values are more than 0.9 for all classifiers.

Assessment of ML Models on ASD Screening Data of Adult

The classification measures achieved by the models on autism data of adult without utilizing any feature selection procedure are represented in Table 4. The NB model outperformed in majority of the measures. This model achieved the accuracy of 97.15% and more than 0.9 value for the remaining measures.

Table 3. Performance measures of ML models with Adolescent Autism data

Performance Measures	Machine Learning Models			
	KNN	**NB**	**SVM**	**DT**
Accuracy (%)	74.19	67.741	61.29	**90.32**
Precision	0.708	0.653	0.612	0.998
Recall	0.944	0.944	0.998	0.833
F-Measure	0.809	0.772	0.76	0.909
AUC	0.958	0.945	0.933	0.974

Table 4. Performance measures of ML models with Adult Autism data

Performance Measures	Machine Learning Models			
	KNN	**NB**	**SVM**	**DT**
Accuracy (%)	86.25	**97.15**	77.41	94.31
Precision	0.723	0.949	0.739	0.901
Recall	0.68	0.949	0.944	0.867
F-Measure	0.701	0.949	0.829	0.884
AUC	0.812	0.997	0.958	0.988

Evaluation of Machine Learning Models With GA based Features

Here, the machine learning models are established using the KNN, NB, SVM and DT classification algorithms by training with the features chosen by the GA based feature selection method. All the three variants of ASD data are involved in training as well testing the ML models.

Assessment of ML Models on ASD Screening Data of Children

The machine learning models are trained with the features selected from the autism data of children using genetic algorithm. The classification measures corresponding to 4 models are depicted in Table 5. The NB classifier performed better for all measures, which is 94.25% for accuracy and greater than 0.9 for remaining measures. The KNN and SVM models achieved comparable values for most of the measures.

Table 5. Performance measures of ML models with GA based features of children autism data

Performance Measures	Machine Learning Models			
	KNN	NB	SVM	DT
Accuracy (%)	87.35	**94.25**	88.5	90.8
Precision	0.886	0.979	0.99	0.954
Recall	0.866	0.904	0.776	0.875
F-Measure	0.876	0.938	0.861	0.913
AUC	0.895	0.985	0.962	0.982

Assessment of ML Models on ASD Screening Data of Adolescent

The classification measures computed for all the models with the subset of features selected from the adolescent autism data are specified in Table 6. The NB and DT models accomplished the best accuracy of 90.32% which is very high compared to the other two models. It also achieved better precision value than the other models. The SVM has shown a variation in the performance measures such as the higher values of recall and AUC measures.

Table 6. Performance measures of ML models with GA based features of adolescent autism data

Performance Measures	Machine Learning Models			
	KNN	NB	SVM	DT
Accuracy (%)	77.41	**90.32**	67.74	**90.32**
Precision	0.708	0.99	0.677	0.985
Recall	0.99	0.812	0.99	0.666
F-Measure	0.829	0.896	0.807	0.8
AUC	0.865	0.987	0.972	0.893

Assessment of ML Models on ASD Screening Data of Adult

The classification measures derived by optimal features selected from the autism data of adult are represented in Table 7. All the ML models attained better accuracy measures (more than 90%) and NB achieved the first position with a value of 97.63%. The AUC scores also more than 0.9 for all the learning models.

Table 7. Performance measures of ML models with GA based features of adult autism data

Performance Measures	Machine Learning Models			
	KNN	NB	SVM	DT
Accuracy (%)	94.78	**97.63**	90.99	94.31
Precision	0.882	0.909	0.944	0.868
Recall	0.9	0.99	0.666	0.929
F-Measure	0.891	0.952	0.781	0.898
AUC	0.931	0.998	0.974	0.98

Evaluation of Machine Learning Models With BTLBO Based Features

Here, the machine learning models are structured by training the KNN, NB, SVM and DT classification algorithms with the features chosen by the BTLBO based feature selection method. The performance of ML models are tested with all the variants of autism data.

Assessment of ML Models on ASD Screening Data of Children

The learning models are trained with the autism data of children using BTLBO algorithm. The classification measures corresponding to 4 models are depicted in Table 8. All ML models performed better for all classification measures, which is 98.855% for accuracy and greater than 0.9 for remaining cases.

Table 8. Performance measures of ML models with BTLBO based features of children autism data

Performance Measures	Machine Learning Models			
	KNN	NB	SVM	DT
Accuracy (%)	**98.85**	**98.85**	**98.85**	96.55
Precision	0.998	0.998	0.977	0.959
Recall	0.978	0.978	0.998	0.979
F-Measure	0.989	0.989	0.988	0.969
AUC	0.999	0.997	0.999	0.986

Assessment of ML Models on ASD Screening Data of Adolescent

The classification measures calculated for all the models with the subset of features selected from the adolescent autism data are specified in Table 9. The SVM and DT models accomplished the best accuracy of 96.77% which is better than the other two models. All 4 models attained better values (more than 0.9) for the remaining measures.

Table 9. Performance measures of ML models with BTLBO based features of Adolescent Autism data

Performance Measures	Machine Learning Models			
	KNN	NB	SVM	DT
Accuracy (%)	90.32	93.54	**96.77**	**96.77**
Precision	0.857	0.9	0.99	0.947
Recall	0.99	0.99	0.947	0.997
F-Measure	0.923	0.947	0.99	0.972
AUC	0.978	0.976	0.995	0.991

Assessment of ML Models on ASD Screening Data of Adult

The classification measures achieved by the features chosen from the autism data of adult individuals are represented in Table 10. All the ML models attained better accuracy measures (more than 90%). Both NB and SVM achieved 99.05% with the selected group of features. The remaining measures are more than 0.9 for all the learning models.

Table 10. Performance measures of ML models with BTLBO based features of Adult Autism data

Performance Measures	Machine Learning Models			
	KNN	NB	SVM	DT
Accuracy (%)	98.57	**99.05**	**99.05**	96.68
Precision	0.96	0.961	0.99	0.942
Recall	0.98	0.99	0.96	0.924
F-Measure	0.97	0.98	0.979	0.933
AUC	0.998	0.998	0.998	0.991

Comparison of ML Models Performance Based on Feature Selection Methods

Moreover, the performance measures accomplished by the machine learning models (KNN, NB, SVM and DT) with respect to complete feature set and optimal subgroup of features are compared using graph illustrations. The optimal subset of features is chosen with the help of GA and BTLBO algorithms. The ROC curves also plotted between false positive rates and true positive rates for classifiers with complete features and BTLBO selected features.

Analogy of ML Models Based on ASD Screening Data of Children

The classification accuracies achieved by the ML models with 3 groups of features are shown in Figure 5. The KNN classifier achieved the significant improvement with GA and BTLBO selected features. There is no change or nominal improvement with NB and SVM models for GA based features and minimal improvement with BTLBO features. The NB model attained the best average classification accuracy (95.78%) in all cases.

Figure 5. Comparison of ML models accuracy on children autism data

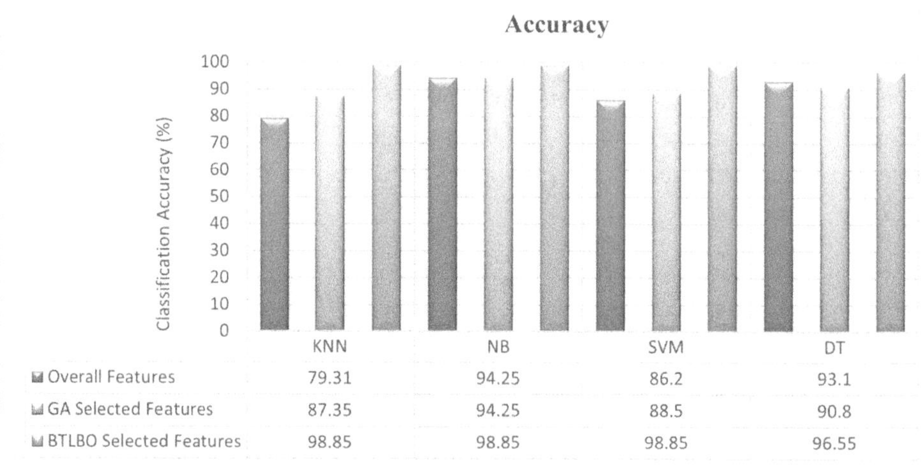

	KNN	NB	SVM	DT
Overall Features	79.31	94.25	86.2	93.1
GA Selected Features	87.35	94.25	88.5	90.8
BTLBO Selected Features	98.85	98.85	98.85	96.55

Figure 6. Comparison of ML models precision and recall values on children autism data

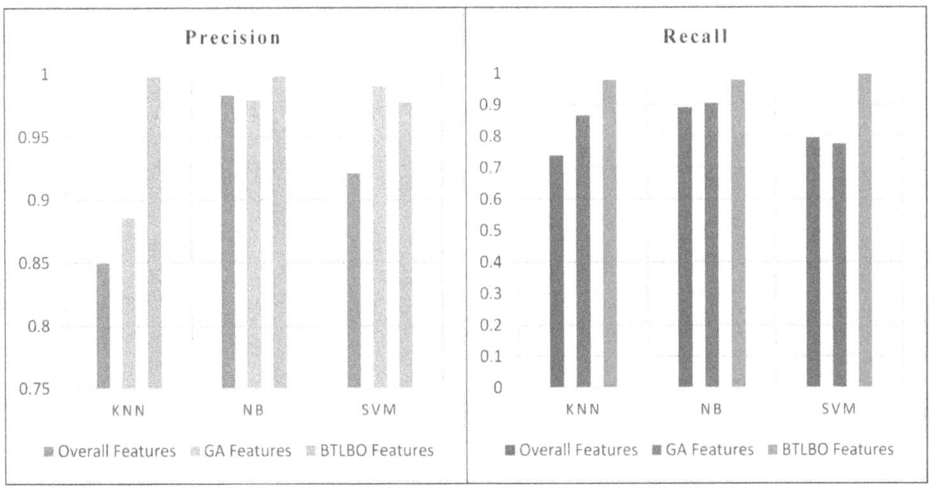

The precision and recall measures are compared for all ML models in terms of bar charts shown in Figure 6. The SVM model achieved improvement for the precision value with the features chosen using optimization algorithms. The features opted by BTLBO algorithm attained maximum improvement for precision value than GA features and original features. The NB model achieved best average precision value in all the three cases. The SVM model attained best recall value with BTLBO features. The NB model achieved best average value with all categories of features. The KNN model derived incremental recall value from original features to GA features and BTLBO features. The comparison of F-Measure and AUC scores are illustrated in charts as shown in Figure 7. The BTLBO model achieved better F-Measure and AUC values for all the ML models. The GA based features attained comparable results with all features of the data. The KNN model achieved better AUC values than the remaining two cases.

The curves plotted for the AUC values of the classifiers with respect to the features of BTLBO and original features are represented in Figure 8. The X-Axis specifies False Positive Rates and Y-Axis specifies True Positive rates of the classifier. The BTLBO based features have provided much difference in the area covered by the curve for KNN classifier. The ROC curves of NB and SVM models are nominally separated in both cases.

Figure 7. Comparison of ML models F-Measure and AUC values on children autism data

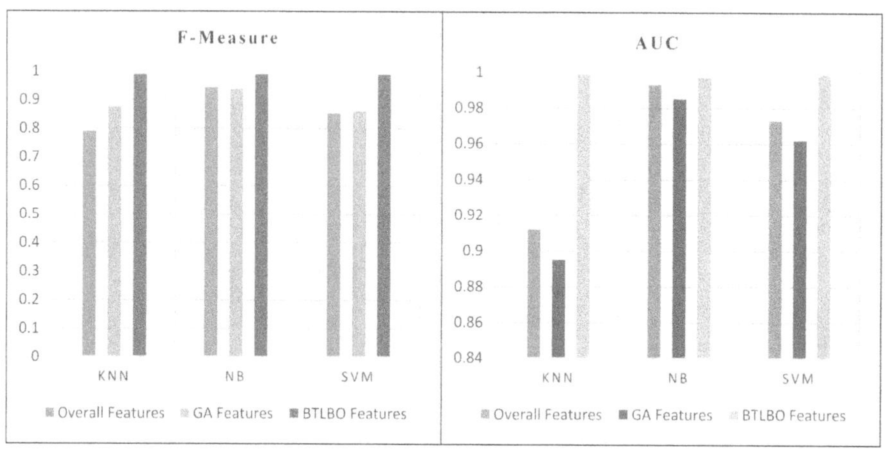

Figure 8. Comparison of ML models ROC curves on children autism data

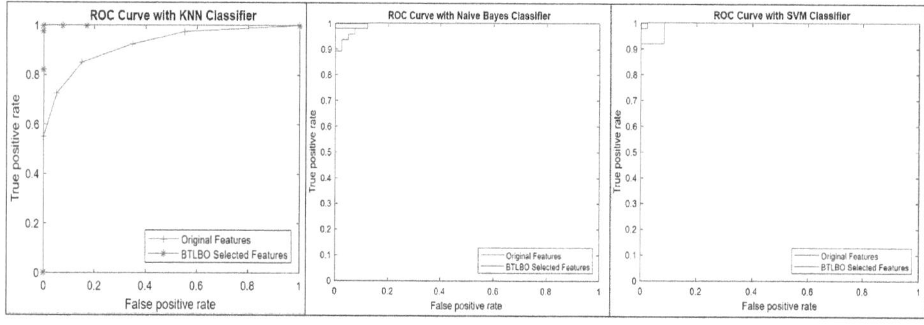

Analogy of ML Models Based on ASD Screening Data of Adolescent

The classification accuracies accomplished by the ML models with 3 categories of features are demonstrated in Figure 9. The SVM and DT models achieved a significant improvement in the accuracy (96.77%) with BTLBO selected features. A nominal improvement has been observed for KNN classifier with GA selected features and better improvement in accuracy with BTLBO selected features. The NB model accomplished better accuracy values with the features opted by the optimization algorithms. The BTLBO based features achieved more than 90% accuracy values with the KNN, NB, SVM and DT models. All ML models attained an average of 81.44% accuracy with GA based features and 93.54% accuracy with BTLBO based features.

Figure 9. Comparison of ML models accuracy on adolescent autism data

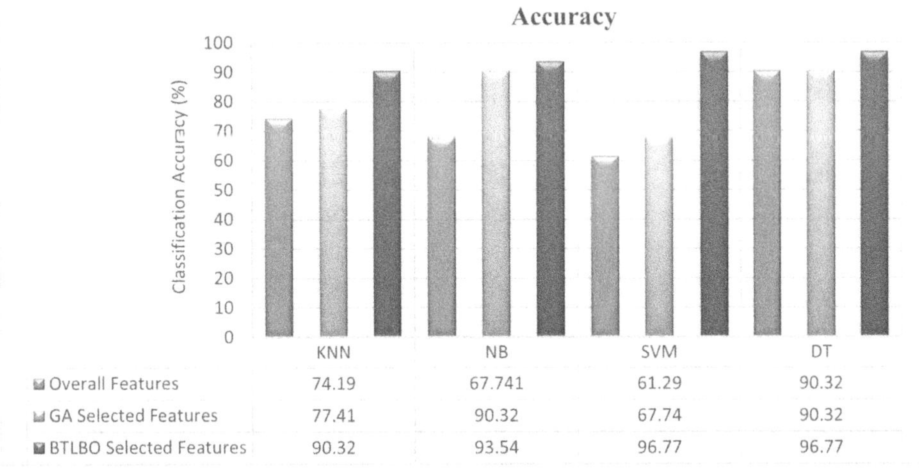

Figure 10. Comparison of ML models precision and recall values on adolescent autism data

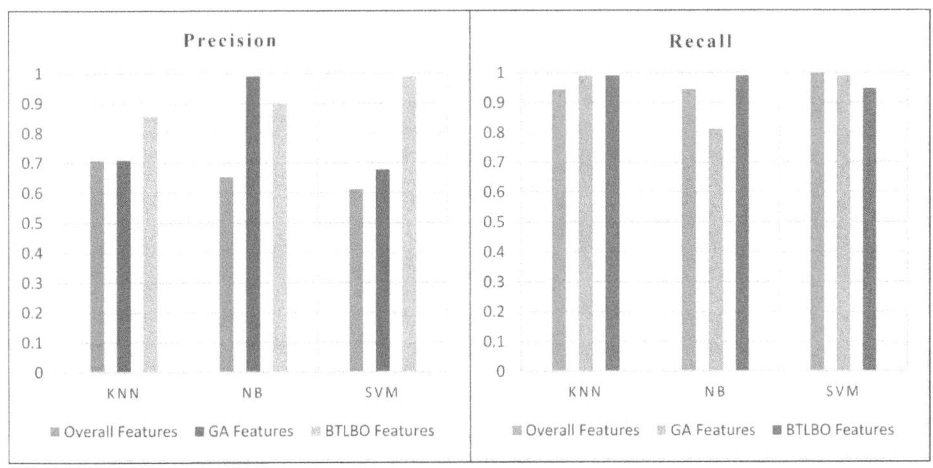

The precision and recall values of the ML models are compared using the charts illustrated in Figure 10. The NB model achieved better performance for the precision value with the features chosen using optimization algorithms. The features selected by BTLBO algorithm attained maximum improvement for the precision value than GA features and original features using KNN and SVM models. The KNN and SVM models attained better recall (more than 0.9) values with complete features as well as the features chosen by the optimization algorithms. The NB model derived incremental recall values from original to BTLBO features except for GA features. The F-Measure and AUC scores are compared using bar charts as specified in Figure 11. The BTLBO model achieved better F-Measure and AUC values for all the ML models. The GA based features achieved minimal improvement for the measures compared to the initial features of the data. All ML models attained similar results except for KNN using GA based features.

The curves plotted for the AUC values of the ML models with respect to the adolescent features chosen by BTLBO algorithm and original features are represented in Figure 12. The BTLBO based features have produced much variation in the area wrapped by the curve for all the classifiers. The ROC curve of SVM with BTLBO features covered maximum space of the graph.

Figure 11. Comparison of ML models F-Measure and AUC values on adolescent autism data

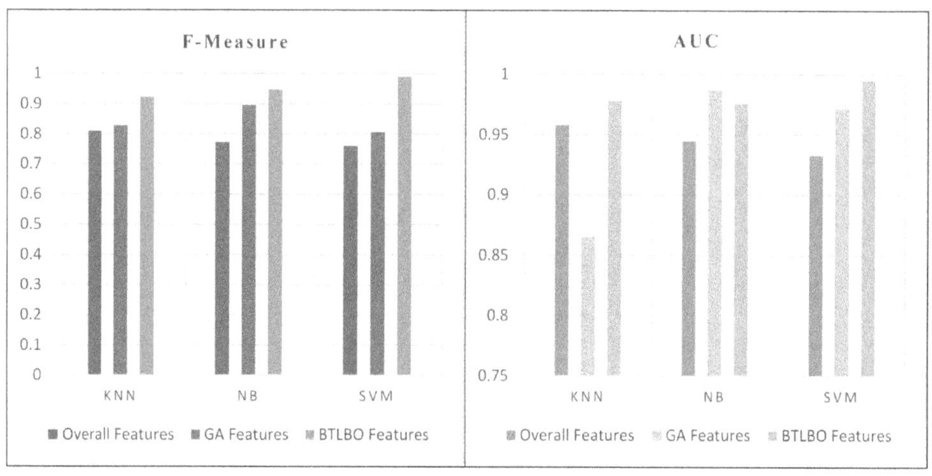

Figure 12. Comparison of ML models ROC curves on adolescent autism data

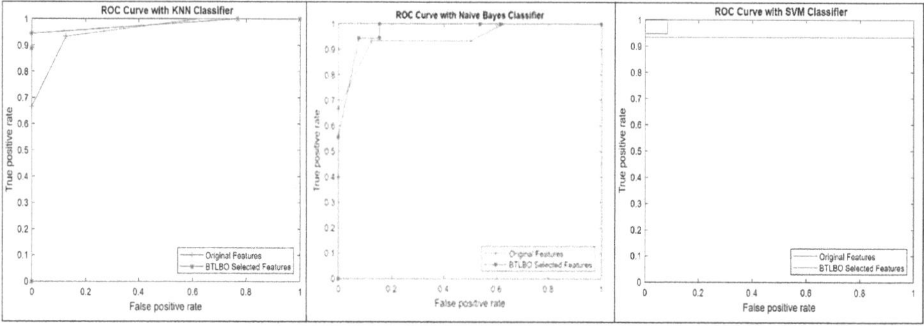

Analogy of ML Models Based on ASD Screening Data of Adult

The classification accuracies achieved by the ML models are compared for the complete feature set and the features chosen by the optimization algorithm on adult autism data. The classification accuracies are specified on y-axis and the classifiers are specified along with the x-axis as shown in Figure 13. The KNN model achieved significant improvement with GA based features in comparison with all features and BTLBO algorithm achieved further improvement in the accuracy. The BTLBO based features accomplished best accuracy value (99.05%) with NB and SVM based models. The NB model attained more than 95% accuracy with all categories of feature sets. The accuracy values of ML models with and without feature selection techniques have proved the importance of optimization algorithms.

The precision and recall measures of ML models are compared with the help of bar charts as displayed in Figure 14. The KNN and SVM models achieved better improvement in the precision values with the features chosen by the GA and BTLBO algorithms. The NB model has attained similar precision and recall values (more than 0.9) for all categories of feature sets. The SVM model achieved best precision value with the feature subsets formed by the optimization algorithms. The KNN model derived incremental precision and recall values from original features to GA based features and BTLBO based features. The comparison of F-Measure and AUC scores of ML models are demonstrated with the help of charts as illustrated in Figure 15. The BTLBO model selected features achieved better F-Measure and AUC values for KNN and SVM models. The NB model attained comparable F-Measure and AUC values with all groups of feature sets.

Figure 13. Comparison of ML models accuracy on adult autism data

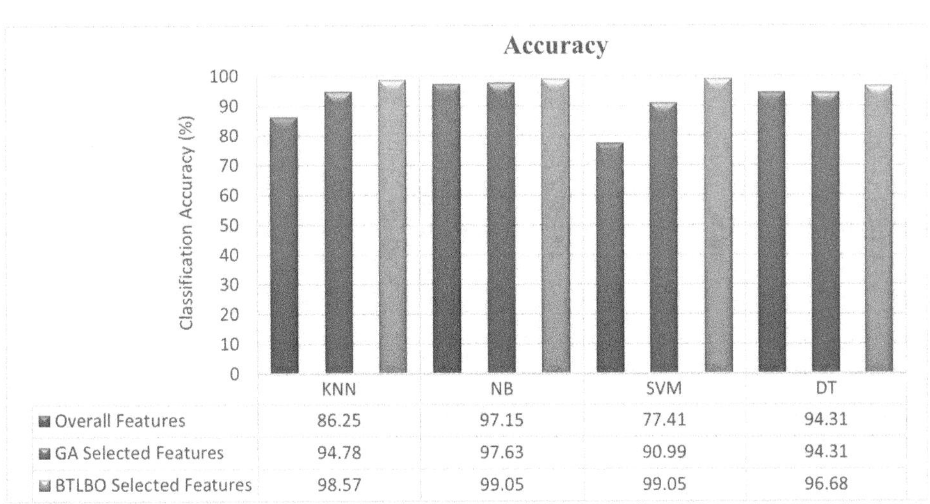

	KNN	NB	SVM	DT
Overall Features	86.25	97.15	77.41	94.31
GA Selected Features	94.78	97.63	90.99	94.31
BTLBO Selected Features	98.57	99.05	99.05	96.68

Figure 14. Comparison of ML models precision and recall values on adult autism data

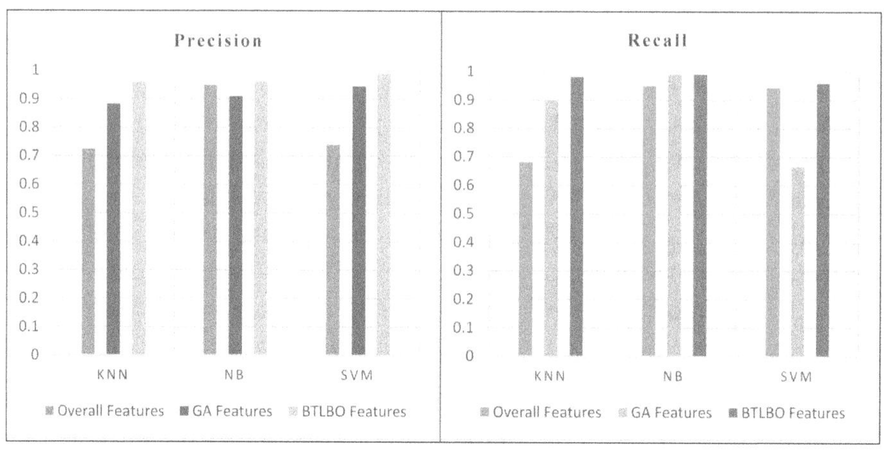

Figure 15. Comparison of ML models F-Measure and AUC values on adult autism data

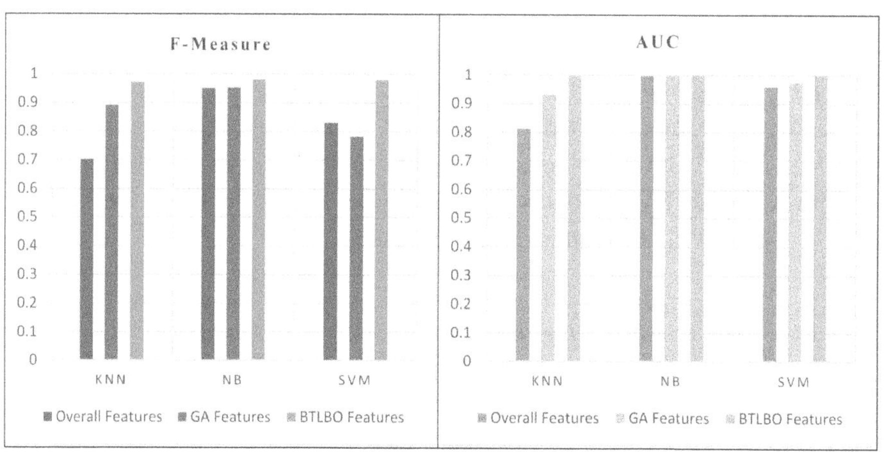

The curves of the graphs shown in the Figure 16 demonstrates the AUC scores attained by the ML models on adult autism data with the complete features and the features of BTLBO algorithm. The BTLBO based features have created significant difference in the area covered by the curves for KNN and SVM classifiers. The ROC curves of NB model are almost overlapped with similar AUC value for complete features set and BTLBO features. The statistics confirmed that the proposed machine learning models performed well with the subset of features chosen by the GA as well as BTLBO algorithms.

Figure 16. Comparison of ML models ROC curves on adult autism data

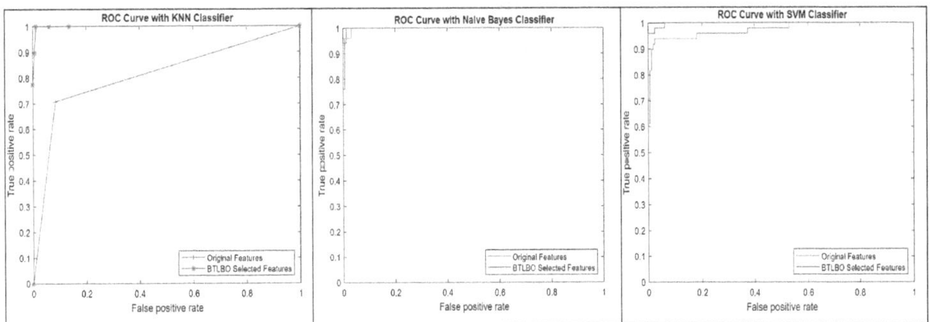

CONCLUSION

In this chapter, several optimized machine learning models are developed with the help evolutionary based feature selection techniques to diagnose the autism in the individuals . The ML models employed well recognized optimization algorithms (GA and BTLBO) for selecting the best combination of subgroup of features from the ASD data of UCI repository. The selected optimal subset of features from the children, adolescent and adult datasets achieved better classification results with KNN, NB, SVM and DT models. The performance measures are compared with the ML models trained with all values of the datasets. These optimized models will help the parents, physicians and experts for early diagnosis of autism in all ages groups of people. . It would be a good choice to perform feature selection with other novel evolutionary optimization algorithms for building machine learning models.

REFERENCES

Adriano, L. I. O., Petronio, L. B., Ricardo, L. M. F., & Márcio, C. (2010). GA-based method for feature selection and parameters optimization for machine learning regression applied to software effort estimation. *Information and Software Technology*, *52*(11), 1155–1166. doi:10.1016/j.infsof.2010.05.009

Allison, C., Auyeung, B., & Baron-Cohen, S. (2012). Toward brief "red flags" for autism screening: The short autism spectrum quotient and the short quantitative checklist for autism in toddlers in 1,000 cases and 3,000 controls. *Journal of the American Academy of Child and Adolescent Psychiatry*, *51*(2), 202–212. doi:10.1016/j.jaac.2011.11.003 PMID:22265366

Baron-Cohen, S., Wheelwright, S., Skinner, R., Martin, J., & Clubley, E. (2001). The autism-spectrum quotient (AQ): Evidence from Asperger syndrome/high-functioning autism, males and females, scientists and mathematicians. *Journal of Autism and Developmental Disorders, 31*(1), 5–17. doi:10.1023/A:1005653411471 PMID:11439754

Cheng-Lung, H., & Chieh-Jen, W. A. (2006). GA-based feature selection and parameters optimization for support vector machines. *Expert Systems with Applications, 31*(2), 231–240. doi:10.1016/j.eswa.2005.09.024

Ender, S., & Tansel, D. (2019). A novel hybrid teaching-learning-based optimization algorithm for the classification of data by using extreme learning machines. *Turkish Journal of Electrical Engineering and Computer Sciences, 27*, 1523–1533.

Fadi, T. (2018). Machine learning in autistic spectrum disorder behavioral research: A review and ways forward. *Informatics for Health & Social Care, 44*, 1–20. PMID:29436887

Hakan, E., Ayça, D., Tansel, D., & Ahmet, C. (2018). Novel multiobjective TLBO algorithms for the feature subset selection problem. *Neurocomputing, 306*, 94–107. doi:10.1016/j.neucom.2018.04.020

Jalaja, J., Geetha, V., & Vivek, R. (2019). Classification of Autism Spectrum Disorder Data using Machine Learning Techniques. *International Journal of Engineering and Advanced Technology, 8*(6S), 565–569. doi:10.35940/ijeat.F1114.0886S19

Kaur, R., & Kautish, S. (2019). Multimodal sentiment analysis: A survey and comparison. *International Journal of Service Science, Management, Engineering, and Technology, 10*(2), 38–58. doi:10.4018/IJSSMET.2019040103

Kenneth, D. J. (1988). Learning with genetic algorithms: An overview. *Machine Learning, 3*(2-3), 121–138. doi:10.1007/BF00113894

Mohamed, A., Nabil, A., & Karma, M. F. (2021). Applying machine learning on home videos for remote autism diagnosis: Further study and analysis. *Health Informatics Journal, 27*(1), 1–13. PMID:33583277

Mohan, A., & Nandhini, M. (2017). A Study on Optimization Techniques in Feature Selection for Medical Image Analysis. *International Journal on Computer Science and Engineering, 9*(3), 75–82.

Mohan, A., & Nandhini, M. (2018). Feature optimization using teaching learning based optimization for breast disease diagnosis. *International Journal of Recent Technology and Engineering, 7*(4), 78–85.

Mohan, A., & Nandhini, M. (2020). Wrapper based Feature Selection using Integrative Teaching Learning Based Optimization Algorithm. *The International Arab Journal of Information Technology*, *17*(6), 885–894. doi:10.34028/iajit/17/6/7

Mohan, A., & Nandhini, M. (in press). Optimal feature selection using binary teaching learning based optimization algorithm. *Journal of King Saud University – Computer and Information Sciences*.

Mythili, M. S., & Mohamed, S. A. R. (2015). A New Hybrid Algorithm for Detecting Autistic children learning skills. *IACSIT International Journal of Engineering and Technology*, *7*(4), 1505–1513.

Nadire, C., & Abdulmalik, A. (2021). A Systematic Literature Review on the Application of Machine-Learning Models in Behavioral Assessment of Autism Spectrum Disorder. *Journal of Personalized Medicine*, *11*(4), 299. doi:10.3390/jpm11040299 PMID:33919878

Rani, S., & Kautish, S. (2018). Application of data mining techniques for prediction of diabetes-A review. International Journal of Scientific Research in Computer Science. *Engineering and Information Technology*, *3*(3), 1996–2004.

Rani, S., & Kautish, S. (2018, June). Association clustering and time series based data mining in continuous data for diabetes prediction. In *2018 second international conference on intelligent computing and control systems (ICICCS)* (pp. 1209-1214). IEEE. 10.1109/ICCONS.2018.8662909

Reyana, A., & Kautish, S. (2021). *Corona virus-related Disease Pandemic: A Review on Machine Learning Approaches and Treatment Trials on Diagnosed Population for Future Clinical Decision Support*. Current Medical Imaging.

Reyana, A., Krishnaprasath, V. T., Kautish, S., Panigrahi, R., & Shaik, M. (2020). Decision-making on the existence of soft exudates in diabetic retinopathy. *International Journal of Computer Applications in Technology*, *64*(4), 375–381. doi:10.1504/IJCAT.2020.112684

Saeid, A. T., Mohammad, R. A., Behzad, Z. D., & Sayed, A. M. (2012). Nonlinear Feature Transformation and Genetic Feature Selection: Improving System Security and Decreasing Computational Cost. *ETRI Journal*, *34*(6), 847–857. doi:10.4218/etrij.12.1812.0032

Sampathkumar, A., Rastogi, R., Arukonda, S., Shankar, A., Kautish, S., & Sivaram, M. (2020). An efficient hybrid methodology for detection of cancer-causing gene using CSC for micro array data. *Journal of Ambient Intelligence and Humanized Computing*, *11*(11), 4743–4751. doi:10.100712652-020-01731-7

Shouheng, T., Longquan, Y., Fang'an, D., Yanhai, L., Yong, L., & Qiuju, L. (2017). HSTLBO: A hybrid algorithm based on Harmony Search and Teaching-Learning Based Optimization for complex high dimensional optimization problems. *PLoS One*, 12. PMID:28403224

Suman, R., & Sarfaraz, M. (2020). Analysis and Detection of Autism Spectrum Disorder Using Machine Learning Techniques. *Procedia Computer Science*, *167*, 994–1004. doi:10.1016/j.procs.2020.03.399

Suresh, C. S., Anima, N., & Parvathi, K. (2013). Rough set and teaching learning based optimization technique for optimal features selection. *Central European Journal of Computer Science*, *3*(1), 27–42.

Thabtah, F. (2017). *ASDTests. A mobile app for ASD screening.* http://asdtests.com

Thabtah, F. (2017). Autism Spectrum Disorder Screening: Machine Learning Adaptation and DSM-5 Fulfillment. *Proceedings of the 1st International Conference on Medical and Health Informatics*, 1-6. 10.1145/3107514.3107515

Thabtah, F. (in press). Machine Learning in Autistic Spectrum Disorder Behavioural Research: A Review. *Informatics for Health and Social Care Journal.*

Ugur, E., & Dang, N. H. T. (2019). Autism Spectrum Disorder Detection with Machine Learning Methods. *Current Psychiatry Research and Reviews*, *15*, 297–308.

Compilation of References

ABC News. (2012, Aug). *Non-verbal girl with Autism speaks through her computer.* https://www.youtube.com/watch?v=xMBzJleeOno

Abrams, M., & Saunders, Z. (2018). Teacher for Children with Autism. *Mechanical Engineering (New York, N.Y.), 140*(12), 35. doi:10.1115/1.2018-DEC-4

Adriano, L. I. O., Petronio, L. B., Ricardo, L. M. F., & Márcio, C. (2010). GA-based method for feature selection and parameters optimization for machine learning regression applied to software effort estimation. *Information and Software Technology, 52*(11), 1155–1166. doi:10.1016/j.infsof.2010.05.009

Akshay, L. C. (2018, Oct). *Mouse Cursor Control Using Facial Movements—An HCI Application.* https://towardsdatascience.com/mouse-control-facial-movements-hci-app-c16b0494a971

Alakwaa, F. M., Chaudhary, K., & Garmire, L. X. (2018). Deep learning accurately predicts estrogen receptor status in breast cancer metabolomics data. *Journal of Proteome Research, 17*(1), 337–347. doi:10.1021/acs.jproteome.7b00595 PMID:29110491

Allison, C., Auyeung, B., & Baron-Cohen, S. (2012). Toward brief "red flags" for autism screening: The short autism spectrum quotient and the short quantitative checklist in 1,000 cases and 3,000 controls. *Journal of the American Academy of Child and Adolescent Psychiatry, 51*(2), 202–212. doi:10.1016/j.jaac.2011.11.003 PMID:22265366

Alpay Savasan, Z., Yilmaz, A., Ugur, Z., Aydas, B., Bahado Singh, R. O., & Graham, S. F. (2019). Metabolomic profiling of cerebral palsy brain tissue reveals nove lcentral biomarkers and biochemical path ways associated with the disease: A pilot study. *Metabolites*, 9. PMID:30717353

Altorok, N., Tsou, P. S., Coit, P., Khanna, D., & Sawalha, A. H. (2014). *Genomewide DNA methylation analysis in dermal fibroblasts from patients with diffuse and limited systemic sclerosis reveals common and subset specific DNA methylation aberrancies. In Diagnostic and Statistical Manual of Mental Disorders (5th ed.).* American Psychiatric Association.

Amaral, C., Mouga, S., Simões, M., Pereira, H.C., Bernardino, I., Quental, H., Playle, R., McNamara, R., Oliveira, G., & Castelo-Branco, M. (2018, July). A Feasibility Clinical Trial to Improve Social Attention in Autistic Spectrum Disorder (ASD) Using a Brain Computer Interface. *Front Neurosci., 13*(12), 477. doi:10.3389/fnins.2018.00477

Aniket Eknath Kudale. (2015, Aug). *Animouse*. https://github.com/aniketkudale/Animouse

Anitha, A., Nakamura, K., Thanseem, I., Yamada, K., Iwayama, Y., Toyota, T., Matsuzaki, H., Miyachi, T., Yamada, S., Tsujii, M., Tsuchiya, K. J., Matsumoto, K., Iwata, Y., Suzuki, K., Ichikawa, H., Sugiyama, T., Yoshikawa, T., & Mori, N. (2012). Brain region -specific altered expression and association of mitochondria related genesinautism. *Molecular Autism*, *3*(1), 12. doi:10.1186/2040-2392-3-12 PMID:23116158

Armstrong, C. (2008). AA Preleases guidelines on identification of children with autism spectrum disorders. *American Family Physician*, *78*, 1301–1305.

Association, A. P. (1994). Diagnostic and Statistical Manual of Mental Disorders (4th ed.). Washington, DC: Author.

Asthana, A., Marks, T. K., Jones, M. J., Tieu, K. H., & Rohith, M. V. (2011, November). Fully automatic pose-invariant face recognition via 3D pose normalization. In *2011 International Conference on Computer Vision* (pp. 937-944). IEEE. 10.1109/ICCV.2011.6126336

Athanaselis, T., Bakamidis, S., Dologlou, I., Argyriou, E. N., & Symvonis, A. (2011). Incorporating Speech Recognition Engine into an Intelligent Assistive Reading System for Dyslexic Students. *Twelfth Annual Conference of the International Speech Communication Association.*

Athanaselis, T., Bakamidis, S., Dologlou, I., Argyriou, E. N., & Symvonis, A. (2014). Making assistive reading tools user friendly: A new platform for Greek dyslexic students empowered by automatic speech recognition. *Multimedia Tools and Applications*, *68*(3), 681–699. doi:10.100711042-012-1073-5

Bahado-Singh, R.O., Yilmaz, A., Bisgin, H., Turkoglu, O., Kumar, P., Sherman, E., Mrazik, A., Odibo, A., & Graham, S.F. (2019). Artificial intelligence and the analysis of multiplatform metabolomics data for the detection of intrauterine growth restriction. *PLoS One, 14.*

Bahado-Singh, R.O., Yilmaz, A., Bisgin, H., Turkoglu, O., Kumar, P., Sherman, E., Mrazik, A., Odibo, A., & Graham, S.F., (2019). Artificial intelligence and the analysis of multi-platform metabolomics data for the detection of intrauterine growth restriction. *PLoS One, 14.*

Bahado-Singh, R. O., Sonek, J., McKenna, D., Cool, D., Aydas, B., Turkoglu, O., Bjorndahl, T., Mandal, R., Wishart, D., Friedman, P., Graham, S. F., & Yilmaz, A. (2018). Artificial Intelligence and amniotic fluid multiomics analysis: The prediction of perinatal outcome in a symptomatic short cervix. *Ultrasound in Obstetrics & Gynecology.*

Bahado-Singh, R. O., Vishweswaraiah, S., Aydas, B., Mishra, N. K., Guda, C., & Radhakrishna, U. (2019). Deep learning / artificial intelligence and blood-based DNA epigenomic prediction of cerebralpalsy. *International Journal of Molecular Sciences*, 20. PMID:31035542

Baron-Cohen, S., Wheelwright, S., Skinner, R., Martin, J., & Clubley, E. (2001). The autism-spectrum quotient (AQ): Evidence from Asperger syndrome/high-functioning autism, males and females, scientists and mathematicians. *Journal of Autism and Developmental Disorders*, *31*(1), 5–17. doi:10.1023/A:1005653411471 PMID:11439754

Basak, S. (2017, Feb) Mouse control with gesture. *Ishara - Mouse Control with Gesture.* https://github.com/saikatbsk/Ishara#readme

Behavior Imaging Solutions. (n.d.). *The Remote Autism Assessment Platform: NODA.* https://www.nodaautismdiagnosis.com/

Bekerom, B. (2017). Using machine learning for detection of autism spectrum disorder. In *Proc. 20th Student Conf. IT* (pp. 1-7). Academic Press.

Bender, L., Goldschmidt, L., Sankar, D. V. S., & Freedman, A. M. (1962). Treatment of Autistic Schizophrenic Children with LSD-25 and UML-491. In J. Wortis (Ed.), *Recent Advances in Biological Psychiatry.* Springer. doi:10.1007/978-1-4684-8306-2_17

Bengio, Y. (2009). Learning deep architectures for AI. Found. Trends®. *Machine Learning, 2*(1), 1–127. doi:10.1561/2200000006

Benjamini, Y., & Hochberg, Y. (1995). Controlling the false discovery rate: A practical and powerful approach to multiple testing. *Journal of the Royal Statistical Society. Series B. Methodological, 57*(1), 289–300. doi:10.1111/j.2517-6161.1995.tb02031.x

Berg, T., & Belhumeur, P. N. (2012, September). Tom-vs-Pete Classifiers and Identity-Preserving Alignment for Face Verification. In BMVC (Vol. 2, p. 7). doi:10.5244/C.26.129

Black, M. H., Chen, N. T. M., Iyer, K. K., Lipp, O. V., Bölte, S., Falkmer, M., Tan, T., & Girdler, S. (2017). Mechanisms of facial emotion recognition in autism spectrum disorders: Insights from eye tracking and electroencephalography. *Neuroscience and Biobehavioral Reviews, 80*, 488–515. doi:10.1016/j.neubiorev.2017.06.016 PMID:28698082

Bone, D., Bishop, S. L., Black, M. P., Goodwin, M. S., Lord, C., & Narayanan, S. S. (2016). Use of machine learning to improve autism screening and diagnostic instruments: Effectiveness, efficiency, and multi-instrument fusion. *Journal of Child Psychology and Psychiatry, and Allied Disciplines, 57*(8), 927–937. doi:10.1111/jcpp.12559 PMID:27090613

Bone, D., Goodwin, M. S., Black, M. P., Lee, C. C., Audhkhasi, K., & Narayanan, S. (2015). Applying machine learning to facilitate autism diagnostics: Pitfalls and promises. *Journal of Autism and Developmental Disorders, 45*(5), 1121–1136. doi:10.100710803-014-2268-6 PMID:25294649

Bone, D., Lee, C. C., Black, M. P., Williams, M. E., Lee, S., Levitt, P., & Narayanan, S. (2014). The psychologist as an interlocutor in autism spectrum disorder assessment: Insights from a study of spontaneous prosody. *Journal of Speech, Language, and Hearing Research: JSLHR, 57*(4), 1162–1177. doi:10.1044/2014_JSLHR-S-13-0062 PMID:24686340

Buescher, A. V., Cidav, Z., Knapp, M., & Mandell, D. S. (2014, August). Costs of autism spectrum disorders in the United Kingdom and the United States. *JAMA Pediatrics, 168*(8), 721–728. doi:10.1001/jamapediatrics.2014.210 PMID:24911948

Butler, M. G., Rafi, S. K., Hossain, W., Stephan, D. A., & Manzardo, A. M. (2015). Whole exome sequencing in females with autism implicates novel and candidate genes. *International Journal of Molecular Sciences, 16*(1), 1312–1335. doi:10.3390/ijms16011312 PMID:25574603

Cao, C., Hou, Q., & Zhou, K. (2014). Displaced dynamic expression regression for real-time facial tracking and animation. *ACM Transactions on Graphics*, *33*(4), 1–10. doi:10.1145/3450626.3459806

Cao, X., Wei, Y., Wen, F., & Sun, J. (2014). Face alignment by explicit shape regression. *International Journal of Computer Vision*, *107*(2), 177–190. doi:10.100711263-013-0667-3

CDC. (2020, Feb). *Screening and Diagnosis of Autism Spectrum Disorder for Healthcare Providers.* https://www.cdc.gov/ncbddd/autism/hcp-screening.html

Cheng-Lung, H., & Chieh-Jen, W. A. (2006). GA-based feature selection and parameters optimization for support vector machines. *Expert Systems with Applications*, *31*(2), 231–240. doi:10.1016/j.eswa.2005.09.024

Chen, Y. A., Lemire, M., Choufani, S., Butcher, D. T., Grafodatskaya, D., Zanke, B. W., Gallinger, S., Hudson, T. J., & Weksberg, R. (2013). Discovery of cross-reactive probes and polymorphic CpGs in the Illumina Infinium Human Methylation 450 microarray. *Epigenetics*, *8*(2), 203–209. doi:10.4161/epi.23470 PMID:23314698

Cognoa. (n.d.). https://cognoa.com/

Constantino, J. N., Lavesser, P. D., Zhang, Y. I., Abbacchi, A. M., Gray, T., & Todd, R. D. (2007). Rapid quantitative assessment of autistic social impairment by classroom teachers. *Journal of the American Academy of Child and Adolescent Psychiatry*, *46*(12), 1668–1676. doi:10.1097/chi.0b013e318157cb23 PMID:18030089

Cootes, T. F., Edwards, G. J., & Taylor, C. J. (2001, June). Active appearance models. *IEEE Transactions on Pattern Analysis and Machine Intelligence*, *23*(6), 681–685. doi:10.1109/34.927467

Cootes, T. F., Taylor, C. J., Cooper, D. H., & Graham, J. (1995). Active shape models-their training and application. *Computer Vision and Image Understanding*, *61*(1), 38–59. doi:10.1006/cviu.1995.1004

CREA Software Systems. (n.d.). *EVA Facial Mouse PRO.* https://play.google.com/store/apps/details?id=com.crea_si.eva_facial_mouse

Cruz, J. A., & Wishart, D. S. (2006). Applications of machine learning in cancer prediction and prognosis. *Cancer Informatics*, *2*. doi:10.1177/117693510600200030 PMID:19458758

Cuschieri, T., Khaled, R., Farrugia, V. E., Martinez, H. P., & Yannakakis, G. N. (2014, September). The iLearnRW game: support for students with Dyslexia in class and at home. In *2014 6th International Conference on Games and Virtual Worlds for Serious Applications (VS-GAMES)* (pp. 1-2). IEEE.

Davenport, T., & Kalakota, R. (2019, June). The potential for artificial intelligence in healthcare. *Future Healthcare Journal*, *6*(2), 94–98. doi:10.7861/futurehosp.6-2-94 PMID:31363513

Del Coco, M., Leo, M., Carcagni, P., Fama, F., Spadaro, L., Ruta, L., Pioggia, G., & Distante, C. (2018). Study of Mechanisms of Social Interaction Stimulation in Autism Spectrum Disorder by Assisted Humanoid Robot. *IEEE Transactions on Cognitive and Developmental Systems*, *10*(4), 993–1004. doi:10.1109/TCDS.2017.2783684

Dhiman, G. (2019b). *Multi-objective Metaheuristic Approaches for Data Clustering in Engineering Application (s)* (Doctoral dissertation).

Dhiman, G., & Kaur, A. (2017, December). Spotted hyena optimizer for solving engineering design problems. In *2017 international conference on machine learning and data science (MLDS)* (pp. 114-119). IEEE.

Dhiman, G. (2019a). ESA: A hybrid bio-inspired metaheuristic optimization approach for engineering problems. *Engineering with Computers*, 1–31. doi:10.100700366-019-00826-w

Dhiman, G. (2020). MOSHEPO: A hybrid multi-objective approach to solve economic load dispatch and micro grid problems. *Applied Intelligence*, *50*(1), 119–137. doi:10.100710489-019-01522-4

Dhiman, G., & Kaur, A. (2018). Optimizing the design of air foil and optical buffer problems using spotted hyena optimizer. *Designs*, *2*(3), 28. doi:10.3390/designs2030028

Dhiman, G., & Kaur, A. (2019). A hybrid algorithm based on particle swarm and spotted hyena optimizer for global optimization. In *Soft Computing for Problem Solving* (pp. 599–615). Springer. doi:10.1007/978-981-13-1592-3_47

Dhiman, G., & Kaur, A. (2019). STOA: A bio-inspired based optimization algorithm for industrial engineering problems. *Engineering Applications of Artificial Intelligence*, *82*, 148–174. doi:10.1016/j.engappai.2019.03.021

Dhiman, G., & Kumar, V. (2017). Spotted hyena optimizer: A novel bio-inspired based metaheuristic technique for engineering applications. *Advances in Engineering Software*, *114*, 48–70. doi:10.1016/j.advengsoft.2017.05.014

Dhiman, G., & Kumar, V. (2018). Emperor penguin optimizer: A bio-inspired algorithm for engineering problems. *Knowledge-Based Systems*, *159*, 20–50. doi:10.1016/j.knosys.2018.06.001

Dhiman, G., & Kumar, V. (2018). Multi-objective spotted hyena optimizer: A multi-objective optimization algorithm for engineering problems. *Knowledge-Based Systems*, *150*, 175–197. doi:10.1016/j.knosys.2018.03.011

Dhiman, G., & Kumar, V. (2019). KnRVEA: A hybrid evolutionary algorithm based on knee points and reference vector adaptation strategies for many-objective optimization. *Applied Intelligence*, *49*(7), 2434–2460. doi:10.100710489-018-1365-1

Dhiman, G., & Kumar, V. (2019). Seagull optimization algorithm: Theory and its applications for large-scale industrial engineering problems. *Knowledge-Based Systems*, *165*, 169–196. doi:10.1016/j.knosys.2018.11.024

Dhiman, G., & Kumar, V. (2019). Spotted hyena optimizer for solving complex and non-linear constrained engineering problems. In *Harmony search and nature inspired optimization algorithms* (pp. 857–867). Springer. doi:10.1007/978-981-13-0761-4_81

Dlib. (n.d.). *C ++ Library*. http://dlib.net/

Dollár, P., Welinder, P., & Perona, P. (2010, June). Cascaded pose regression. In *2010 IEEE Computer Society Conference on Computer Vision and Pattern Recognition* (pp. 1078-1085). IEEE.

Duquette, A., Michaud, F., & Mercier, H. (2008). Exploring the use of a mobile robot as an imitation agent with children with low-functioning autism. *Autonomous Robots*, *24*(2), 147–157. doi:10.100710514-007-9056-5

Eisenberg, L. (1957). The fathers of autistic children. *The American Journal of Orthopsychiatry*, *27*(4), 715–724. doi:10.1111/j.1939-0025.1957.tb05539.x PMID:13470021

Elkind, J., Cohen, K., & Murray, C. (1993). Using computer-based readers to improve reading comprehension of students with dyslexia. *Annals of Dyslexia*, *43*(1), 238–259. doi:10.1007/BF02928184 PMID:24233995

Ender, S., & Tansel, D. (2019). A novel hybrid teaching-learning-based optimization algorithm for the classification of data by using extreme learning machines. *Turkish Journal of Electrical Engineering and Computer Sciences*, *27*, 1523–1533.

Eni, M., Dinstein, I., Ilan, M., Menashe, I., Meiri, G., & Zigel, Y. (2020). Estimating Autism Severity in Young Children from Speech Signals Using a Deep Neural Network. *IEEE Access: Practical Innovations, Open Solutions*, *8*, 139489–139500. doi:10.1109/ACCESS.2020.3012532

Fakoor, R., Ladhak, F., Nazi, A., & Huber, M. (2013). Using deep learning to enhance cancer diagnosis and classification. *Proceedings of the ICML Workshop on the Role of Machine Learning in Transforming Healthcare.*

Falconer, J. (2013, May). *Nao Robot Goes to School to Help Kids With Autism.* https://spectrum.ieee.org/automaton/robotics/humanoids/aldebaran-robotics-nao-robot-autism-solution-for-kids

Fernández, A., Usamentiaga, R., Carús, J. L., & Casado, R. (2016). Driver distraction using visual-based sensors and algorithms. *Sensors (Basel)*, *16*(11), 1805. doi:10.339016111805 PMID:27801822

Fridenson-Hayo, S., Berggren, S., Lassalle, A., Tal, S., Pigat, D., Bölte, S., Baron-Cohen, S., & Golan, O. (2016). Basic and complex emotion recognition in children with autism: Cross-cultural findings. *Molecular Autism*, *7*(1), 1–11. doi:10.118613229-016-0113-9 PMID:28018573

Girli, A., Doğmaz, S., & Fakültesi, E. (2018). Ability of Children with Learning Disabilities and Children with Autism Spectrum Disorder to Recognize Feelings from Facial Expressions and Body Language. *World J Educ*, *8*(2), 10. Advance online publication. doi:10.5430/wje.v8n2p10

Goyal, S. B., Bedi, P., Kumar, J., & Varadarajan, V. (2021). Deep learning application for sensing available spectrum for cognitive radio: An ECRNN approach. *Peer-to-Peer Networking and Applications*. Advance online publication. doi:10.100712083-021-01169-4

Hagen, A., Pellom, B., Van Vuuren, S., & Cole, R. (2004). Advances in children's speech recognition within an interactive literacy tutor. In *Proceedings of HLT-NAACL 2004: Short Papers* (pp. 25-28). 10.3115/1613984.1613991

Hakan, E., Ayça, D., Tansel, D., & Ahmet, C. (2018). Novel multiobjective TLBO algorithms for the feature subset selection problem. *Neurocomputing*, *306*, 94–107. doi:10.1016/j.neucom.2018.04.020

Hanson, D., Mazzei, D., Garver, C., Ahluwalia, A., De Rossi, D., Stevenson, M., & Reynolds, K. (2012, June). Realistic humanlike robots for treatment of ASD, social training, and research; shown to appeal to youths with ASD, cause physiological arousal, and increase human-to-human social engagement. *Proceedings of the 5th ACM international conference on pervasive technologies related to assistive environments (PETRA'12).*

Hardesty, L. (2018, Apr). *Computer system transcribes words users "speak silently"*. https://news.mit.edu/2018/computer-system-transcribes-words-users-speak-silently-0404#:~:text=MIT%20researchers%20have%20developed%20a,does%20not%20actually%20speak%20aloud.&text=The%20signals%20are%20fed%20to,particular%20signals%20with%20particular%20words

Hauck, F., & Kliewer, N. (2017). Machine Learning for Autism Diagnostics: Applying Support Vector Classification. *Int'l Conf. Health Informatics and Medical Systems.*

Heinsfeld, A. S., Franco, A. R., Craddock, R. C., Buchweitz, A., & Meneguzzi, F. (2018). Identification of autism spectrum disorder using deep learning and the ABIDE dataset. *NeuroImage. Clinical*, *17*, 16–23. doi:10.1016/j.nicl.2017.08.017 PMID:29034163

Hockey, G. R. J., Hockey, R., Gaillard, A. W., & Burov, O. (Eds.). (2003). *Operator functional state: the assessment and prediction of human performance degradation in complex tasks* (Vol. 355). IOS Press.

Huang, G. B., & Learned-Miller, E. (2014). *Labeled faces in the wild: Updates and new reporting procedures.* Dept. Comput. Sci., Univ. Massachusetts Amherst, *Tech. Rep*, *14*(003).

Husni, H. (2012). Automatic transcription of dyslexic children-s read speech. *Global Journal on Technology*, 2.

Husni, H., & Jamaluddin, Z. (2008, October). A retrospective and future look at speech recognition applications in assisting children with reading disabilities. *Proceedings of the world Congress on Engineering and Computer Science.*

Husni, H., & Jamaludin, Z. (2009). ASR Technology for Children with Dyslexia: Enabling Immediate Intervention to Support Reading in Bahasa Melayu. *Online Submission*, *6*(6), 64–70.

Hu, Y., Jiang, D., Yan, S., & Zhang, L. (2004, May). Automatic 3D reconstruction for face recognition. In *Sixth IEEE International Conference on Automatic Face and Gesture Recognition, 2004. Proceedings.* (pp. 843-848). IEEE.

Instruments, O. (n.d.). *HeadMouse® Nano Wireless Head Controlled Access Works on Computers, Smartphones, Tablets – Everything!* https://www.orin.com/access/headmouse/#:~:text=HeadMouse%20replaces%20the%20standard%20computer,the%20mouse%20pointer%20follows%20along

Irani, A., Moradi, H., & Vahid, L. K. (2018). Autism Screening Using a Video Game Based on Emotions. In *2018 2nd National and 1st International Digital Games Research Conference: Trends, Technologies, and Applications, DGRC 2018*. Institute of Electrical and Electronics Engineers Inc. 10.1109/DGRC.2018.8712053

Islam, J., Mubassira, M., Islam, M. R., & Das, A. K. (2019, February). A speech recognition system for Bengali language using recurrent Neural network. In *2019 IEEE 4th international conference on computer and communication systems (ICCCS)* (pp. 73-76). IEEE.

Jalaja, J., Geetha, V., & Vivek, R. (2019). Classification of Autism Spectrum Disorder Data using Machine Learning Techniques. *International Journal of Engineering and Advanced Technology*, *8*(6S), 565–569. doi:10.35940/ijeat.F1114.0886S19

Jayawardana, Y., Jaime, M., & Jayarathna, S. (2019). Analysis of temporal relationships between ASD and brain activity through EEG and machine learning. In *Proceedings - 2019 IEEE 20th International Conference on Information Reuse and Integration for Data Science, IRI 2019*. Institute of Electrical and Electronics Engineers Inc. 10.1109/IRI.2019.00035

John, G. H., & Langley, P. (2013). *Estimating continuous distributions in Bayesian classifiers*. arXiv preprint arXiv:1302.4964.

Kamath & Dalwai. (2017, May). IAP Chapter of Neuro Developmental Pediatrics. *National Guidelines Autism.*

Kaur, K., & Pany, S. (2017). Computer-based intervention for autism spectrum disorder children and their social skills: A meta-analysis. *Scholarly Research Journal for Humanity Science & English Language.*, *4*(23). Advance online publication. doi:10.21922rjhsel.v4i23.9649

Kaur, R., & Kautish, S. (2019). Multimodal sentiment analysis: A survey and comparison. *International Journal of Service Science, Management, Engineering, and Technology*, *10*(2), 38–58. doi:10.4018/IJSSMET.2019040103

Kautish, S., & Ahmed, R. K. A. (2016). A Comprehensive Review of Current and Future Applications of Data Mining in Medicine & Healthcare. *Algorithms*, *6*(8), 9.

Kazemi, V., & Sullivan, J. (2014). One millisecond face alignment with an ensemble of regression trees. *2014 IEEE Conference on Computer Vision and Pattern Recognition*, 1867-1874. 10.1109/CVPR.2014.241

Keerthi, S. S., Shevade, S. K., Bhattacharyya, C., & Murthy, K. R. K. (2001). Improvements to Platt's SMO algorithm for SVM classifier design. *Neural Computation*, *13*(3), 637–649. doi:10.1162/089976601300014493

Ke, F., Choi, S., Kang, Y. H., Cheon, K.-A., & Lee, S. W. (2020). Exploring the Structural and Strategic Bases of Autism Spectrum Disorders with Deep Learning. *IEEE Access: Practical Innovations, Open Solutions*, *8*, 153341–153352. doi:10.1109/ACCESS.2020.3016734

Ke, F., & Yang, R. (2020). Classification and Biomarker Exploration of Autism Spectrum Disorders Based on Recurrent Attention Model. *IEEE Access: Practical Innovations, Open Solutions*, *8*, 216298–216307. doi:10.1109/ACCESS.2020.3038479

Kenneth, D. J. (1988). Learning with genetic algorithms: An overview. *Machine Learning*, *3*(2-3), 121–138. doi:10.1007/BF00113894

Khakhar, J., & Madhvanath, S. (2010, November). Jollymate: Assistive technology for young children with dyslexia. In *2010 12th International Conference on Frontiers in Handwriting Recognition* (pp. 576-580). IEEE.

Khan, N. S., Muaz, M. H., Kabir, A., & Islam, M. N. (2017, December). Diabetes predicting mhealth application using machine learning. In *2017 IEEE International WIE Conference on Electrical and Computer Engineering (WIECON-ECE)* (pp. 237-240). IEEE. 10.1109/WIECON-ECE.2017.8468885

Kosmicki, J. A., Sochat, V., Duda, M., & Wall, D. P. (2015). Searching for a minimal set of behaviors for autism detection through feature selection-based machine learning. *Translational Psychiatry*, *5*(2), e514–e514. doi:10.1038/tp.2015.7 PMID:25710120

Kozima, H., Michalowski, M. P., & Nakagawa, C. (2009). Keepon. *International Journal of Social Robotics*, *1*(1), 3–18. doi:10.100712369-008-0009-8

Lanka, P., Rangaprakash, D., Dretsch, M. N., Katz, J. S., Denney, T. S. Jr, & Deshpande, G. (2020). Supervised machine learning for diagnostic classification from large-scale neuroimaging datasets. *Brain Imaging and Behavior*, *14*(6), 2378–2416. doi:10.100711682-019-00191-8 PMID:31691160

Lefkovits, S., Lefkovits, L., & Emerich, S. (2017, April). Detecting the eye and its openness with Gabor filters. In *2017 5th International Symposium on Digital Forensic and Security (ISDFS)* (pp. 1-5). IEEE. 10.1109/ISDFS.2017.7916506

Li, G., Chen, M. H., Li, G., Wu, D., Lian, C., Sun, Q., Shen, D., & Wang, L. (2019). A Longitudinal MRI Study of Amygdala and Hippocampal Subfields for Infants with Risk of Autism. Lecture Notes in Computer Science (Including Subseries Lecture Notes in Artificial Intelligence and Lecture Notes in Bioinformatics), 11849, 164–171. doi:10.1007/978-3-030-35817-4_20

Li, X., Dvornek, N. C., & Papademetris, X. (2018) 2-Channel convolutional 3D deep neural network (2CC3D) for fMRI analysis: ASD classification and feature learning. In *Proceedings - International Symposium on Biomedical Imaging*. IEEE Computer Society.

Liaw, A., & Wiener, M. (2002). Classification and regression by random Forest. *R News*, *2*(3), 18–22.

Li, B., Sharma, A., Meng, J., Purushwalkam, S., & Gowen, E. (2017). Applying machine learning to identify autistic adults using imitation: An exploratory study. *PLoS One*, *12*(8), e0182652. doi:10.1371/journal.pone.0182652 PMID:28813454

List of Files. (n.d.). http://dlib.net/files

Liu, B., Ma, Y., & Wong, C. K. (2001). Classification using association rules: weaknesses and enhancements. In *Data mining for scientific and engineering applications* (pp. 591–605). Springer. doi:10.1007/978-1-4615-1733-7_30

Liu, W., Li, M., & Yi, L. (2016). Identifying children with autism spectrum disorder based on their face processing abnormality: A machine learning framework. *Autism Research*, *9*(8), 888–898. doi:10.1002/aur.1615 PMID:27037971

Matsuda, S., Minagawa, Y., & Yamamoto, J. (2015). Gaze Behavior of Children with ASD toward Pictures of Facial Expressions. Autism Research and Treatment. doi:10.1155/2015/617190

Mihajlović, S., Kupusinac, A., Ivetić, D., & Berković, I. (2020). *The Use of Python in the field of Artificial Intelligence*. Academic Press.

Mohamed, A., Nabil, A., & Karma, M. F. (2021). Applying machine learning on home videos for remote autism diagnosis: Further study and analysis. *Health Informatics Journal*, *27*(1), 1–13. PMID:33583277

Mohan, A., & Nandhini, M. (in press). Optimal feature selection using binary teaching learning based optimization algorithm. *Journal of King Saud University – Computer and Information Sciences*.

Mohan, A., & Nandhini, M. (2017). A Study on Optimization Techniques in Feature Selection for Medical Image Analysis. *International Journal on Computer Science and Engineering*, *9*(3), 75–82.

Mohan, A., & Nandhini, M. (2018). Feature optimization using teaching learning based optimization for breast disease diagnosis. *International Journal of Recent Technology and Engineering*, *7*(4), 78–85.

Mohan, A., & Nandhini, M. (2020). Wrapper based Feature Selection using Integrative Teaching Learning Based Optimization Algorithm. *The International Arab Journal of Information Technology*, *17*(6), 885–894. doi:10.34028/iajit/17/6/7

Moon, S. J., Hwang, J., Kana, R., Torous, J., & Kim, J. W. (2019). Accuracy of machine learning algorithms for the diagnosis of autism spectrum disorder: Systematic review and meta-analysis of brain magnetic resonance imaging studies. Journal of Medical Internet Research, 21(12). doi:10.2196/14108

Moreno, C. (2018). Use of HCI for the development of emotional skills in the treatment of Autism Spectrum Disorder. *Systematic Reviews*, 1–6. doi:10.23919/CISTI.2018.8399209

Mostafa, S., Tang, L., & Wu, F. X. (2019). Diagnosis of Autism Spectrum Disorder Based on Eigenvalues of Brain Networks. *IEEE Access: Practical Innovations, Open Solutions*, *7*, 128474–128486. doi:10.1109/ACCESS.2019.2940198

Mouse, S. (n.d.). https://smylemouse.com/

Mythili, M. S., & Mohamed, S. A. R. (2015). A New Hybrid Algorithm for Detecting Autistic children learning skills. *IACSIT International Journal of Engineering and Technology*, *7*(4), 1505–1513.

Mythili, M. S., & Shanavas, A. M. (2014). A study on Autism spectrum disorders using classification techniques. *International Journal of Soft Computing and Engineering*, *4*(5), 88–91.

Nadire, C., & Abdulmalik, A. (2021). A Systematic Literature Review on the Application of Machine-Learning Models in Behavioral Assessment of Autism Spectrum Disorder. *Journal of Personalized Medicine*, *11*(4), 299. doi:10.3390/jpm11040299 PMID:33919878

National Autistic Society. (2020, Aug). *Employing autistic people – a guide for employers.* https://www.autism.org.uk/advice-and-guidance/topics/employment/employing-autistic-people/employers

Newman, J. (2014, Oct). *To Siri, With Love.* https://www.nytimes.com/2014/10/19/fashion/how-apples-siri-became-one-autistic-boys-bff.html

Omar, K. S., Mondal, P., Khan, N. S., Rizvi, M. R. K., & Islam, M. N. (2019). A machine learning approach to predict autism spectrum disorder. In *2019 International Conference on Electrical, Computer and Communication Engineering (ECCE)* (pp. 1-6). IEEE. 10.1109/ECACE.2019.8679454

Ouherrou, N., Elhammoumi, O., Benmarrakchi, F., & El Kafi, J. (2018, October). A heuristic evaluation of an educational game for children with dyslexia. In *2018 IEEE 5th International Congress on Information Science and Technology (CiSt)* (pp. 386-390). IEEE.

Ozdenizci, O., Cumpanasoiu, C., Mazefsky, C., Siegel, M., Erdogmus, D., & Ioannidis, S. (2018). *Time-series prediction of proximal aggression on set in minimally-verbal youth with autism spectrum disorder using physiological biosignals.* arXiv:1809.09948.

Pace, G. M., Iwata, B. A., Edwards, G. L., & McCosh, K. C. (1986). Stimulus fading and transfer in the treatment of self-restraint and self-injurious behavior. *Journal of Applied Behavior Analysis*, *19*(4), 381–389. doi:10.1901/jaba.1986.19-381 PMID:3804871

Parsons. (2018, July). *The costs of autism strap many families.* Orlando Sentinels. https://www.orlandosentinel.com/health/get-healthy-orlando/os-families-cost-of-autism-20180702-story.html

Pelios, L., Morren, J., Tesch, D., & Axelrod, S. (1999). The impact of functional analysis methodology on treatment choice for self-injurious and aggressive behavior. *Journal of Applied Behavior Analysis*, *32*(2), 185–195. doi:10.1901/jaba.1999.32-185 PMID:10396771

Plötz, T., Hammerla, N. Y., & Olivier, P. (2011). Feature learning for activity recognition in ubiquitous computing. *IJCAI Proceedings-International Joint Conference on Artificial Intelligence.*

Plötz, T., Hammerla, N. Y., Rozga, A., Reavis, A., Call, N., & Abowd, G. D. (2012). Automatic assessment of problem behavior in individuals with developmental disabilities. Paper presented at the proceedings of the 2012 ACM conference on ubiquitous computing. 10.1145/2370216.2370276

Poliker, R. (2006). Pattern recognition. In *Wiley Encyclopedia of biomedical engineering*. Wiley. doi:10.1002/9780471740360.ebs0904

Preece, S. J., Goulermas, J. Y., Kenney, L. P., Howard, D., Meijer, K., & Crompton, R. (2009). Activity identification using body-mounted sensors - A review of classification techniques. *Physiological Measurement*, *30*(4), R1–R33. doi:10.1088/0967-3334/30/4/R01 PMID:19342767

Pugliese, C. E., Kenworthy, L., Bal, V. H., Wallace, G. L., Yerys, B.E., & Maddox, B. B. (2015). Replication and comparison of the newly proposed ADOS-2, module 4 algorithm in ASD without ID: A multi-site study. *Journal of Autism and Developmental Disorders, 45*(12), 3919–3931. . doi:10.100710803-015-2586-3

Rad, N. M., Furlanello, C., & Kessler, F. B. (2016). Applying deep learning to stereo typical motor movement detection in autism spectrum disorders. *2016 IEEE 16th international conference on data mining workshops*.

Rahman, F. A., Mokhtar, F., Alias, N. A., & Saleh, R. (2012). Multimedia elements as instructions for dyslexic children. *International Journal of Education and Information Technologies*, *6*(2), 193–200.

Raj, S., & Masood, S. (2020). Analysis and Detection of Autism Spectrum Disorder Using Machine Learning Techniques. In *Procedia Computer Science* (pp. 994–1004). Elsevier B.V. doi:10.1016/j.procs.2020.03.399

Ramdoss, S., Lang, R., Mulloy, A., Franco, J., O'Reilly, M., Didden, R., & Lancioni, G. (2011). Use of Computer-Based Interventions to Teach Communication Skills to Children with Autism Spectrum Disorders: A Systematic Review. *Journal of Behavioral Education*, *20*(1), 55–76. doi:10.100710864-010-9112-7

Rani, S., & Kautish, S. (2018, June). Association clustering and time series based data mining in continuous data for diabetes prediction. In *2018 second international conference on intelligent computing and control systems (ICICCS)* (pp. 1209-1214). IEEE. 10.1109/ICCONS.2018.8662909

Rani, S., & Kautish, S. (2018). Application of data mining techniques for prediction of diabetes-A review. International Journal of Scientific Research in Computer Science. *Engineering and Information Technology*, *3*(3), 1996–2004.

Raskind, M. H., & Higgins, E. L. (1999). Speaking to read: The effects of speech recognition technology on the reading and spelling performance of children with learning disabilities. *Annals of Dyslexia*, *49*(1), 251–281. doi:10.100711881-999-0026-9

Rello, L., Bayarri, C., Otal, Y., & Pielot, M. (2014, October). A computer-based method to improve the spelling of children with dyslexia. In *Proceedings of the 16th international ACM SIGACCESS conference on Computers & accessibility* (pp. 153-160). ACM.

Ren, S., Cao, X., Wei, Y., & Sun, J. (2016). Face alignment via regressing local binary features. *IEEE Transactions on Image Processing*, *25*(3), 1233–1245. doi:10.1109/TIP.2016.2518867 PMID:26800539

Reyana, A., & Kautish, S. (2021). *Corona virus-related Disease Pandemic: A Review on Machine Learning Approaches and Treatment Trials on Diagnosed Population for Future Clinical Decision Support*. Current Medical Imaging.

Reyana, A., Krishnaprasath, V. T., Kautish, S., Panigrahi, R., & Shaik, M. (2020). Decision-making on the existence of soft exudates in diabetic retinopathy. *International Journal of Computer Applications in Technology*, *64*(4), 375–381. doi:10.1504/IJCAT.2020.112684

Robokind. (n.d.). *A non-threatening way for learners with ASD to practice their communication and social skills*. https://www.robokind.com/robots4autism/meet-milo

Rosebrock. (2017a, Apr). *Eye blink detection with OpenCV, Python, and dlib*. Academic Press.

Rosebrock. (2017b, Apr). *Detect eyes, nose, lips, and jaw with dlib, OpenCV, and Python*. Academic Press.

Rusli, N., Sidek, S. N., Yusof, H. M., Ishak, N. I., Khalid, M., & Dzulkarnain, A. A. A. (2020). Implementation of Wavelet Analysis on Thermal Images for Affective States Recognition of Children with Autism Spectrum Disorder. *IEEE Access: Practical Innovations, Open Solutions*, *8*, 120818–120834. doi:10.1109/ACCESS.2020.3006004

Russell, M., Brown, C., Skilling, A., Series, R., Wallace, J., Bonham, B., & Barker, P. (1996, October). Applications of automatic speech recognition to speech and language development in young children. In *Proceeding of Fourth International Conference on Spoken Language Processing. ICSLP'96* (Vol. 1, pp. 176-179). IEEE. 10.1109/ICSLP.1996.607069

Sadouk, L., Gadi, T., & Essoufi, E. H. (2018). A Novel Deep Learning Approach for Recognizing Stereotypical Motor Movements within and across Subjects on the Autism Spectrum Disorder. *Computational Intelligence and Neuroscience*, *2018*, 1–16. Advance online publication. doi:10.1155/2018/7186762 PMID:30111994

Saeid, A. T., Mohammad, R. A., Behzad, Z. D., & Sayed, A. M. (2012). Nonlinear Feature Transformation and Genetic Feature Selection: Improving System Security and Decreasing Computational Cost. *ETRI Journal*, *34*(6), 847–857. doi:10.4218/etrij.12.1812.0032

Sagonas, C., Antonakos, E., Tzimiropoulos, G., Zafeiriou, S., & Pantic, M. (2016). 300 faces in-the-wild challenge: Database and results. *Image and Vision Computing*, *47*, 3–18. doi:10.1016/j.imavis.2016.01.002

Sagonas, C., Tzimiropoulos, G., Zafeiriou, S., & Pantic, M. (2013). 300 faces in-the-wild challenge: The first facial landmark localization challenge. In *Proceedings of the IEEE International Conference on Computer Vision Workshops* (pp. 397-403). 10.1109/ICCVW.2013.59

Sagonas, C., Tzimiropoulos, G., Zafeiriou, S., & Pantic, M. (2013). A semi-automatic methodology for facial landmark annotation. In *Proceedings of the IEEE conference on computer vision and pattern recognition workshops* (pp. 896-903). 10.1109/CVPRW.2013.132

Saini, G. K., Chouhan, H., Kori, S., Gupta, A., Shabaz, M., Jagota, V., & Singh, B. K. (2021). Recognition of Human Sentiment from Image using Machine Learning. *Annals of the Romanian Society for Cell Biology*, *25*(5), 1802–1808.

Sampathkumar, A., Rastogi, R., Arukonda, S., Shankar, A., Kautish, S., & Sivaram, M. (2020). An efficient hybrid methodology for detection of cancer-causing gene using CSC for micro array data. *Journal of Ambient Intelligence and Humanized Computing*, *11*(11), 4743–4751. doi:10.100712652-020-01731-7

Santhoshkumar, & Kalaiselvi Geetha. (2019). Emotion Recognition System for Autism Children using Non-verbal Communication. *International Journal of Innovative Technology and Exploring Engineering*, *8*(8), 159-165.

Saputra, M. R. U., & Risqi, M. (2015). LexiPal: Design, implementation and evaluation of gamification on learning application for dyslexia. *International Journal of Computers and Applications*, *131*(7), 37–43. doi:10.5120/ijca2015907416

Schenkman, L. (2020, August). *Motor difficulties in autism, explained*. https://www.spectrumnews.org/news/motor-difficulties-in-autism-explained/

Schmidt, A. P., & Schneider, M. (2007, September). Adaptive Reading Assistance for Dyslexic Students: Closing the Loop. In LWA (pp. 389-391). Academic Press.

Schwartz, O. (2019, Oct). *Mind-reading tech? How private companies could gain access to our brains*. https://www.theguardian.com/technology/2019/oct/24/mind-reading-tech-private-companies-access-brains#:~:text=A%20BCI%20is%20a%20device,be%20recognized%20by%20the%20machine

Sharma, S. R., Gonda, X., & Tarazi, F. I. (2018, May). Autism Spectrum Disorder: Classification, diagnosis and therapy. *Pharmacology & Therapeutics*, *190*, 91–104. Advance online publication. doi:10.1016/j.pharmthera.2018.05.007 PMID:29763648

Sherkatghanad, Z., Akhondzadeh, M., Salari, S., Zomorodi-Moghadam, M., Abdar, M., Acharya, U. R., Khosrowabadi, R., & Salari, V. (2020). Automated Detection of Autism Spectrum Disorder Using a Convolutional Neural Network. *Frontiers in Neuroscience*, *13*, 1325. doi:10.3389/fnins.2019.01325 PMID:32009868

Shouheng, T., Longquan, Y., Fang'an, D., Yanhai, L., Yong, L., & Qiuju, L. (2017). HSTLBO: A hybrid algorithm based on Harmony Search and Teaching-Learning Based Optimization for complex high dimensional optimization problems. *PLoS One*, 12. PMID:28403224

Sigafoos, J., Green, V. A., Edrisinha, C., & Lancioni, G. E. (2007). Flashback to the 1960s: LSD in the treatment of autism. *Developmental Neurorehabilitation*, *10*(1), 75–81. doi:10.1080/13638490601106277 PMID:17608329

Singh, A., Chandewar, C., & Pattarkine, P. (2018). Driver drowsiness alert system with effective feature extraction. *Int. JR in Emer. Sciences et Techniques (Paris)*, *5*(4), 26–31.

Singh, P., & Dhiman, G. (2017, December). A fuzzy-LP approach in time series forecasting. In *International Conference on Pattern Recognition and Machine Intelligence* (pp. 243-253). Springer. 10.1007/978-3-319-69900-4_31

Singh, P., & Dhiman, G. (2018). A hybrid fuzzy time series forecasting model based on granular computing and bio-inspired optimization approaches. *Journal of Computational Science*, *27*, 370–385. doi:10.1016/j.jocs.2018.05.008

Singh, P., & Dhiman, G. (2018). Uncertainty representation using fuzzy-entropy approach: Special application in remotely sensed high-resolution satellite images (RSHRSIs). *Applied Soft Computing*, *72*, 121–139. doi:10.1016/j.asoc.2018.07.038

Sixty-Seventh World Health Assembly Geneva. (2014, May). *WHA67.8: Comprehensive and coordinated efforts for the management of autism spectrum disorders*. Palais des Nations.

Smith, V., & Sung, A. (2014). Computer Interventions for ASD. In V. Patel, V. Preedy, & C. Martin (Eds.), *Comprehensive Guide to Autism*. Springer., doi:10.1007/978-1-4614-4788-7_134

Soukupova, T., & Cech, J. (2016, February). *Eye blink detection using facial landmarks*. In 21st computer vision winter workshop, Rimske Toplice, Slovenia.

Su, Q., Chen, F., & Li, H. (2019). Multimodal emotion perception in children with autism spectrum disorder by eye tracking study. In *2018 IEEE EMBS Conference on Biomedical Engineering and Sciences, IECBES 2018 - Proceedings*. Institute of Electrical and Electronics Engineers Inc.

Suresh, C. S., Anima, N., & Parvathi, K. (2013). Rough set and teaching learning based optimization technique for optimal features selection. *Central European Journal of Computer Science*, *3*(1), 27–42.

Taileb, M., Al-Saggaf, R., Al-Ghamdi, A., Al-Zebaidi, M., & Al-Sahafi, S. (2013, July). YUSR: Speech recognition software for dyslexics. In *International Conference of Design, User Experience, and Usability* (pp. 296-303). Springer.

Tao, Y., & Shyu, M. L. (2019). SP-ASDNet: CNN-LSTM based ASD classification model using observer scanpaths. In *Proceedings - 2019 IEEE International Conference on Multimedia and Expo Workshops, ICMEW 2019*. Institute of Electrical and Electronics Engineers Inc.

Tapus, A., Peca, A., Aly, A., Pop, C., Jisa, L., Pintea, S., ... David, D. O. (2012). Children with autism social engagement in interaction with Nao, an imitative robot: A series of single case experiments. *Interaction Studies: Social Behaviour and Communication in Biological and Artificial Systems*, *13*(3), 315–347. doi:10.1075/is.13.3.01tap

Thabtah, F. (2017). *ASDTests. A mobile app for ASD screening*. Academic Press.

Thabtah, F. (2017). *ASDTests. A mobile app for ASD screening*. http://asdtests.com

Thabtah, F. F. (2017). *Autistic spectrum disorder screening data for children data set*. Academic Press.

Thabtah, F. (2017). Autism spectrum disorder screening: Machine learning adaptation and DSM-5 fulfillment. *Proceedings of the 1st International Conference on Medical and Health Informatics (MDPI)*, 1–6.

Thabtah, F. (2017). Autism Spectrum Disorder Screening: Machine Learning Adaptation and DSM-5 Fulfillment. *Proceedings of the 1st International Conference on Medical and Health Informatics*, 1-6. 10.1145/3107514.3107515

Thabtah, F. (2019). Machine learning in autistic spectrum disorder behavioral research: A review and ways forward. *Informatics for Health & Social Care*, *44*(3), 278–297. doi:10.1080/17538157.2017.1399132 PMID:29436887

Thabtah, F. (in press). Machine Learning in Autistic Spectrum Disorder Behavioural Research: A Review. *Informatics for Health and Social Care Journal*.

Thabtah, F., Kamalov, F., & Rajab, K. (2018). A new computational intelligence approach to detect autistic features for autism screening. *International Journal of Medical Informatics*, *117*, 112–124. doi:10.1016/j.ijmedinf.2018.06.009 PMID:30032959

Ugur, E., & Dang, N. H. T. (2019). Autism Spectrum Disorder Detection with Machine Learning Methods. *Current Psychiatry Research and Reviews*, *15*, 297–308.

Vahia, V. N. (2013). Diagnostic and statistical manual of mental disorders 5: A quick glance. *Indian Journal of Psychiatry*, *55*(3), 220–223. doi:10.4103/0019-5545.117131 PMID:24082241

Vaishali, R., & Sasikala, R. (2018). A machine learning based approach to classify autism with optimum behaviour sets. *Int. J. Eng. Technol*, *7*, 18.

Viacam, E. (n.d.). https://eviacam.crea-si.com/index.php

Voineagu, I., Wang, X., Johnston, P., Lowe, J.K., Tian, Y., Horvath, S., Mill, J., Cantor, R.M., Blencowe, B.J., & Geschwind, D.H. (2011). Transcriptomic analysis of autistic brain reveals convergent molecular pathology. *Nature, 474*, 380–384.

Voineagu, I., Wang, X., Johnston, P., Lowe, J. K., Tian, Y., Horvath, S., Mill, J., Cantor, R. M., Blencowe, B. J., & Geschwind, D. H. (2011). Transcriptomic analysis of autistic brain reveals convergent molecular pathology. *Nature*, *474*(7351), 380–384. doi:10.1038/nature10110 PMID:21614001

Wainer, J., Robins, B., Amirabdollahian, F., & Dautenhahn, K. (2014, September). Using the Humanoid Robot KASPAR to Autonomously Play Triadic Games and Facilitate Collaborative Play Among Children With Autism. *IEEE Transactions on Autonomous Mental Development*, *6*(3), 183–199. doi:10.1109/TAMD.2014.2303116

Wall, D. P., Dally, R., Luyster, R., Jung, J. Y., & DeLuca, T. F. (2012). Use of artificial intelligence to shorten the behavioral diagnosis of autism. *PLoS One*, *7*(8), e43855. doi:10.1371/journal.pone.0043855 PMID:22952789

Wall, D. P., Kosmicki, J., Deluca, T. F., Harstad, E., & Fusaro, V. A. (2012). Use of machine learning to shorten observation-based screening and diagnosis of autism. *Translational Psychiatry*, *2*(4), e100–e100. doi:10.1038/tp.2012.10 PMID:22832900

Wang, J., Cherkassky, V. L., & Just, M. A. (2017). Predicting the brain activation pattern associated with the propositional content of a sentence: Modeling neural representations of events and states. *Human Brain Mapping*, *38*(10), 4865–4881. doi:10.1002/hbm.23692 PMID:28653794

Wang, L. (2017). Datamining, machine learning and big data analytics. *Int. Trans. Electr. Comput. Eng. Syst.*, *4*, 55–61.

Wang, M., Zhang, D., Huang, J., Yap, P.-T., Shen, D., & Liu, M. (2020). Identifying Autism Spectrum Disorder with Multi-Site fMRI via Low-Rank Domain Adaptation. *IEEE Transactions on Medical Imaging*, *39*(3), 644–655. doi:10.1109/TMI.2019.2933160 PMID:31395542

Wang, X. H., Jiao, Y., & Li, L. (2018). Identifying individuals with attention deficit hyperactivity disorder based on temporal variability of dynamic functional connectivity. *Scientific Reports*, *8*(1), 1–12. doi:10.103841598-018-30308-w PMID:30087369

Wilhelm-Benartzi, C. S., Koestler, D. C., Karagas, M. R., Flanagan, J. M., Christensen, B. C., Kelsey, K. T., Marsit, C. J., Houseman, E. A., & Brown, R. (2013). Review of processing and analysis methods for DNA methylation array data. *British Journal of Cancer*, *109*(6), 1394–1402. doi:10.1038/bjc.2013.496 PMID:23982603

Williams, S. M., Nix, D., & Fairweather, P. (2013, April). Using speech recognition technology to enhance literacy instruction for emerging readers. In *Fourth International Conference of the Learning Sciences* (pp. 115-120). Academic Press.

Winden, K. D., Ebrahimi-Fakhari, D., & Sahin, M. (2018). Abnormal mTOR Activation in Autism. *Annual Review of Neuroscience*, *41*(1), 1–23. doi:10.1146/annurev-neuro-080317-061747 PMID:29490194

Wong, N., Morley, R., Saffery, R., & Craig, J. (2008). Archived Guthrie blood spots as a novel source for quantitative DNA methylation analysis. *Biotechniques, 45*.

Wysa. (n.d.). https://www.wysa.io/

Xiao, Z., Qiu, T., Ke, X., Xiao, X., Xiao, T., Liang, F., Zou, B., Huang, H., Fang, H., Chu, K., Zhang, J., & Liu, Y. (2014). Autism spectrum disorder as early neuro developmental disorder: Evidence from the brain imaging abnormalities in 2–3 years old toddlers. *Journal of Autism and Developmental Disorders*, *44*(7), 1633–1640. doi:10.100710803-014-2033-x PMID:24419870

Xiao, Z., Wu, J., Wang, C., Jia, N., & Yang, X. (2019). Computer-aided diagnosis of school-aged children with ASD using full frequency bands and enhanced SAE: A multi-institution study. *Experimental and Therapeutic Medicine*, *17*(5), 4055. doi:10.3892/etm.2019.7448 PMID:31007742

Xiong, X., & De la Torre, F. (2013). Supervised descent method and its applications to face alignment. In *Proceedings of the IEEE conference on computer vision and pattern recognition* (pp. 532-539). 10.1109/CVPR.2013.75

Yang, X., Shyu, M. L., Yu, H. Q., Sun, S.-M., Yin, N.-S., & Chen, W. (2019). Integrating image and textual information in human–robot interactions for children with autism spectrum disorder. *IEEE Transactions on Multimedia, 21*(3), 746–759. doi:10.1109/TMM.2018.2865828

Yoo, J. H., Kim, J. I., Kim, B. N., & Jeong, B. (2020). Exploring characteristic features of attention-deficit/hyperactivity disorder: Findings from multi-modal MRI and candidate genetic data. *Brain Imaging and Behavior, 14*(6), 2132–2147. doi:10.100711682-019-00164-x PMID:31321662

Zhao, H., Swanson, A. R., Weitlauf, A. S., Warren, Z. E., & Sarkar, N. (2018). Hand-in-Hand: A Communication-Enhancement Collaborative Virtual Reality System for Promoting Social Interaction in Children with Autism Spectrum Disorders. *IEEE Transactions on Human-Machine Systems, 48*(2), 136–148. doi:10.1109/THMS.2018.2791562 PMID:30345182

Zheng, Z., Young, E. M., Swanson, A. R., Weitlauf, A. S., Warren, Z. E., & Sarkar, N. (2016). Robot-Mediated Imitation Skill Training for Children with Autism. *IEEE Transactions on Neural Systems and Rehabilitation Engineering, 24*(6), 682–691. doi:10.1109/TNSRE.2015.2475724 PMID:26353376

Zhu, G., Jiang, B., Tong, L., Xie, Y., Zaharchuk, G., & Wintermark, M. (2019). Applications of deep learning to neuro-imaging techniques. *Frontiers in Neurology, 10*(Aug), 869. doi:10.3389/fneur.2019.00869 PMID:31474928

Zhu, X., Lei, Z., Yan, J., Yi, D., & Li, S. Z. (2015). High-fidelity pose and expression normalization for face recognition in the wild. In *Proceedings of the IEEE conference on computer vision and pattern recognition* (pp. 787-796). IEEE.

Zhu, X., & Ramanan, D. (2012, June). *Face detection, pose estimation, and landmark localization in the wild. In 2012 IEEE conference on computer vision and pattern recognition.* IEEE.

Zwaigenbaum, L., Bauman, M. L., Fein, D., Pierce, K., Buie, T., Davis, P. A., Newschaffer, C., Robins, D. L., Wetherby, A., Choueiri, R., Kasari, C., Stone, W. L., Yirmiya, N., Estes, A., Hansen, R. L., Mc Partland, J. C., Natowicz, M. R., Carter, A., Granpeesheh, D., ... Wagner, S. (2015). Early screening of autism spectrum disorder: Recommendations for practice and research. *Pediatrics, 136*(Suppl1), S41–S59. doi:10.1542/peds.2014-3667D PMID:26430169

Related References

To continue our tradition of advancing information science and technology research, we have compiled a list of recommended IGI Global readings. These references will provide additional information and guidance to further enrich your knowledge and assist you with your own research and future publications.

Abu Seman, S. A., & Ramayah, T. (2017). Are We Ready to App?: A Study on mHealth Apps, Its Future, and Trends in Malaysia Context. In J. Pelet (Ed.), *Mobile Platforms, Design, and Apps for Social Commerce* (pp. 69–83). Hershey, PA: IGI Global. doi:10.4018/978-1-5225-2469-4.ch005

Aggarwal, S., & Azad, V. (2017). A Hybrid System Based on FMM and MLP to Diagnose Heart Disease. In S. Bhattacharyya, S. De, I. Pan, & P. Dutta (Eds.), *Intelligent Multidimensional Data Clustering and Analysis* (pp. 293–325). Hershey, PA: IGI Global. doi:10.4018/978-1-5225-1776-4.ch011

Akaichi, J., & Mhadhbi, L. (2016). A Clinical Decision Support System: Ontology-Driven Approach for Effective Emergency Management. In J. Moon & M. Galea (Eds.), *Improving Health Management through Clinical Decision Support Systems* (pp. 270–294). Hershey, PA: IGI Global. doi:10.4018/978-1-4666-9432-3.ch013

Akerkar, R. (2016). Towards an Intelligent Integrated Approach for Clinical Decision Support. In A. Aggarwal (Ed.), *Managing Big Data Integration in the Public Sector* (pp. 187–205). Hershey, PA: IGI Global. doi:10.4018/978-1-4666-9649-5.ch011

Al-Busaidi, S. S. (2018). Interdisciplinary Relationships Between Medicine and Social Sciences. In M. Al-Suqri, A. Al-Kindi, S. AlKindi, & N. Saleem (Eds.), *Promoting Interdisciplinarity in Knowledge Generation and Problem Solving* (pp. 124–137). Hershey, PA: IGI Global. doi:10.4018/978-1-5225-3878-3.ch009

Al Kareh, T., & Thoumy, M. (2018). The Impact of Health Information Digitization on the Physiotherapist-Patient Relationship: A Pilot Study of the Lebanese Community. *International Journal of Healthcare Information Systems and Informatics, 13*(2), 29–53. doi:10.4018/IJHISI.2018040103

Alenzuela, R. (2017). Research, Leadership, and Resource-Sharing Initiatives: The Role of Local Library Consortia in Access to Medical Information. In S. Ram (Ed.), *Library and Information Services for Bioinformatics Education and Research* (pp. 199–211). Hershey, PA: IGI Global. doi:10.4018/978-1-5225-1871-6.ch012

Ameri, H., Alizadeh, S., & Noughabi, E. A. (2017). Application of Data Mining Techniques in Clinical Decision Making: A Literature Review and Classification. In E. Noughabi, B. Raahemi, A. Albadvi, & B. Far (Eds.), *Handbook of Research on Data Science for Effective Healthcare Practice and Administration* (pp. 257–295). Hershey, PA: IGI Global. doi:10.4018/978-1-5225-2515-8.ch012

Anand, S. (2017). Medical Image Enhancement Using Edge Information-Based Methods. In B. Singh (Ed.), *Computational Tools and Techniques for Biomedical Signal Processing* (pp. 123–148). Hershey, PA: IGI Global. doi:10.4018/978-1-5225-0660-7.ch006

Angjellari-Dajci, F., Sapienza, C., Lawless, W. F., & Kavanagh, K. (2016). Human Capital Accumulation in Medical Simulated Learning Environments: A Framework for Economic Evaluation. In M. Russ (Ed.), *Quantitative Multidisciplinary Approaches in Human Capital and Asset Management* (pp. 65–88). Hershey, PA: IGI Global. doi:10.4018/978-1-4666-9652-5.ch004

Anil, M., Ayyildiz-Tamis, D., Tasdemir, S., Sendemir-Urkmez, A., & Gulce-Iz, S. (2016). Bioinspired Materials and Biocompatibility. In M. Bououdina (Ed.), *Emerging Research on Bioinspired Materials Engineering* (pp. 294–322). Hershey, PA: IGI Global. doi:10.4018/978-1-4666-9811-6.ch011

Anton, J. L., Soriano, J. V., Martinez, M. I., & Garcia, F. B. (2018). Comprehensive E-Learning Appraisal System. In M. Khosrow-Pour, D.B.A. (Ed.), Encyclopedia of Information Science and Technology, Fourth Edition (pp. 5787-5799). Hershey, PA: IGI Global. doi:10.4018/978-1-5225-2255-3.ch503

Arabi, M. (2016). Redesigning the Organizational Structure to Reach Efficiency: The Case of Ministry of Health and Medical Education of Iran. In R. Gholipour & K. Rouzbehani (Eds.), *Social, Economic, and Political Perspectives on Public Health Policy-Making* (pp. 257–294). Hershey, PA: IGI Global. doi:10.4018/978-1-4666-9944-1.ch012

Assis-Hassid, S., Heart, T., Reychav, I., & Pliskin, J. S. (2016). Modelling Factors Affecting Patient-Doctor-Computer Communication in Primary Care. *International Journal of Reliable and Quality E-Healthcare*, *5*(1), 1–17. doi:10.4018/IJRQEH.2016010101

Atzori, B., Hoffman, H. G., Vagnoli, L., Messeri, A., & Grotto, R. L. (2018). Virtual Reality as Distraction Technique for Pain Management in Children and Adolescents. In M. Khosrow-Pour, D.B.A. (Ed.), Encyclopedia of Information Science and Technology, Fourth Edition (pp. 5955-5965). Hershey, PA: IGI Global. doi:10.4018/978-1-5225-2255-3.ch518

Audibert, M., Mathonnat, J., Pélissier, A., & Huang, X. X. (2018). The Impact of the New Rural Cooperative Medical Scheme on Township Hospitals' Utilization and Income Structure in Weifang Prefecture, China. In I. Management Association (Ed.), Health Economics and Healthcare Reform: Breakthroughs in Research and Practice (pp. 109-121). Hershey, PA: IGI Global. doi:10.4018/978-1-5225-3168-5.ch007

Ayyachamy, S. (2016). Analysis and Comparison of Developed 2D Medical Image Database Design using Registration Scheme, Retrieval Scheme, and Bag-of-Visual-Words. In N. Dey & A. Ashour (Eds.), *Classification and Clustering in Biomedical Signal Processing* (pp. 149–168). Hershey, PA: IGI Global. doi:10.4018/978-1-5225-0140-4.ch007

Babalola, A. C. (2016). Literacy and Decision Making on Health Issues among Married Women in Southwest Nigeria. In V. Wang (Ed.), *Handbook of Research on Advancing Health Education through Technology* (pp. 191–212). Hershey, PA: IGI Global. doi:10.4018/978-1-4666-9494-1.ch009

Babu, A., & Ayyappan, S. (2017). A Methodological Evaluation of Crypto-Watermarking System for Medical Images. In C. Bhatt & S. Peddoju (Eds.), *Cloud Computing Systems and Applications in Healthcare* (pp. 189–217). Hershey, PA: IGI Global. doi:10.4018/978-1-5225-1002-4.ch010

Bakke, A. (2017). Ethos in E-Health: From Informational to Interactive Websites. In M. Folk & S. Apostel (Eds.), *Establishing and Evaluating Digital Ethos and Online Credibility* (pp. 85–103). Hershey, PA: IGI Global. doi:10.4018/978-1-5225-1072-7.ch005

Bali, S. (2018). Enhancing the Reach of Health Care Through Telemedicine: Status and New Possibilities in Developing Countries. In U. Pandey & V. Indrakanti (Eds.), *Open and Distance Learning Initiatives for Sustainable Development* (pp. 339–354). Hershey, PA: IGI Global. doi:10.4018/978-1-5225-2621-6.ch019

Barrett, T. E. (2018). Essentials for Education and Training for Tomorrow's Physicians. In C. Smith (Ed.), *Exploring the Pressures of Medical Education From a Mental Health and Wellness Perspective* (pp. 230–252). Hershey, PA: IGI Global. doi:10.4018/978-1-5225-2811-1.ch010

Barrett, T. J. (2016). Knowledge in Action: Fostering Health Education through Technology. In V. Wang (Ed.), *Handbook of Research on Advancing Health Education through Technology* (pp. 39–62). Hershey, PA: IGI Global. doi:10.4018/978-1-4666-9494-1.ch003

Berrahal, S., & Boudriga, N. (2017). The Risks of Wearable Technologies to Individuals and Organizations. In A. Marrington, D. Kerr, & J. Gammack (Eds.), *Managing Security Issues and the Hidden Dangers of Wearable Technologies* (pp. 18–46). Hershey, PA: IGI Global. doi:10.4018/978-1-5225-1016-1.ch002

Bhagat, A. P., & Atique, M. (2016). Medical Image Mining Using Fuzzy Connectedness Image Segmentation: Efficient Retrieval of Patients' Stored Images. In W. Karâa & N. Dey (Eds.), *Biomedical Image Analysis and Mining Techniques for Improved Health Outcomes* (pp. 184–209). Hershey, PA: IGI Global. doi:10.4018/978-1-4666-8811-7.ch009

Bhargava, P. (2018). Blended Learning: An Effective Application to Clinical Teaching. In S. Tang & C. Lim (Eds.), *Preparing the Next Generation of Teachers for 21st Century Education* (pp. 302–320). Hershey, PA: IGI Global. doi:10.4018/978-1-5225-4080-9.ch018

Binh, N. T., & Tuyet, V. T. (2016). The Combination of Adaptive Filters to Improve the Quality of Medical Images in New Wavelet Domain. In N. Dey & A. Ashour (Eds.), *Classification and Clustering in Biomedical Signal Processing* (pp. 46–76). Hershey, PA: IGI Global. doi:10.4018/978-1-5225-0140-4.ch003

Bird, J. L. (2017). Writing Healing Narratives. In V. Bryan & J. Bird (Eds.), *Healthcare Community Synergism between Patients, Practitioners, and Researchers* (pp. 1–28). Hershey, PA: IGI Global. doi:10.4018/978-1-5225-0640-9.ch001

Bottrighi, A., Leonardi, G., Piovesan, L., & Terenziani, P. (2016). Knowledge-Based Support to the Treatment of Exceptions in Computer Interpretable Clinical Guidelines. *International Journal of Knowledge-Based Organizations, 6*(3), 1–27. doi:10.4018/IJKBO.2016070101

Bougoulias, K., Kouris, I., Prasinos, M., Giokas, K., & Koutsouris, D. (2017). Ob/Gyn EMR Software: A Solution for Obstetricians and Gynecologists. In A. Moumtzoglou (Ed.), *Design, Development, and Integration of Reliable Electronic Healthcare Platforms* (pp. 101–111). Hershey, PA: IGI Global. doi:10.4018/978-1-5225-1724-5.ch006

Bouslimi, R., Ayadi, M. G., & Akaichi, J. (2018). Medical Image Retrieval in Healthcare Social Networks. *International Journal of Healthcare Information Systems and Informatics*, *13*(2), 13–28. doi:10.4018/IJHISI.2018040102

Bouzaabia, O., Bouzaabia, R., & Mejri, K. (2017). Role of Internet in the Development of Medical Tourism Service in Tunisia. In A. Capatina & E. Rancati (Eds.), *Key Challenges and Opportunities in Web Entrepreneurship* (pp. 211–241). Hershey, PA: IGI Global. doi:10.4018/978-1-5225-2466-3.ch009

Briz-Ponce, L., Juanes-Méndez, J. A., & García-Peñalvo, F. J. (2016). The Role of Gender in Technology Acceptance for Medical Education. In M. Cruz-Cunha, I. Miranda, R. Martinho, & R. Rijo (Eds.), *Encyclopedia of E-Health and Telemedicine* (pp. 1013–1027). Hershey, PA: IGI Global. doi:10.4018/978-1-4666-9978-6.ch079

Briz-Ponce, L., Juanes-Méndez, J. A., & García-Peñalvo, F. J. (2016). A Research Contribution to the Analysis of Mobile Devices in Higher Education from Medical Students' Point of View. In L. Briz-Ponce, J. Juanes-Méndez, & F. García-Peñalvo (Eds.), *Handbook of Research on Mobile Devices and Applications in Higher Education Settings* (pp. 196–221). Hershey, PA: IGI Global. doi:10.4018/978-1-5225-0256-2.ch009

Brown-Jackson, K. L. (2018). Telemedicine and Telehealth: Academics Engaging the Community in a Call to Action. In S. Burton (Ed.), *Engaged Scholarship and Civic Responsibility in Higher Education* (pp. 166–193). Hershey, PA: IGI Global. doi:10.4018/978-1-5225-3649-9.ch008

Bwalya, K. J. (2017). Next Wave of Tele-Medicine: Virtual Presence of Medical Personnel. In K. Moahi, K. Bwalya, & P. Sebina (Eds.), *Health Information Systems and the Advancement of Medical Practice in Developing Countries* (pp. 168–180). Hershey, PA: IGI Global. doi:10.4018/978-1-5225-2262-1.ch010

Carlton, E. L., Holsinger, J. W. Jr, & Anunobi, N. (2016). Physician Engagement with Health Information Technology: Implications for Practice and Professionalism. *International Journal of Computers in Clinical Practice*, *1*(2), 51–73. doi:10.4018/IJCCP.2016070103

Castillo-Page, L., Eliason, J., Conrad, S. S., & Nivet, M. A. (2016). Diversity in Undergraduate Medical Education: An Examination of Organizational Culture and Climate in Medical Schools. In C. Scott & J. Sims (Eds.), *Developing Workforce Diversity Programs, Curriculum, and Degrees in Higher Education* (pp. 304–326). Hershey, PA: IGI Global. doi:10.4018/978-1-5225-0209-8.ch016

Cebeci, H. I., & Hiziroglu, A. (2016). Review of Business Intelligence and Intelligent Systems in Healthcare Domain. In N. Celebi (Ed.), *Intelligent Techniques for Data Analysis in Diverse Settings* (pp. 192–206). Hershey, PA: IGI Global. doi:10.4018/978-1-5225-0075-9.ch009

Celik, G. (2018). Determining Headache Diseases With Genetic Algorithm. In U. Kose, G. Guraksin, & O. Deperlioglu (Eds.), *Nature-Inspired Intelligent Techniques for Solving Biomedical Engineering Problems* (pp. 249–262). Hershey, PA: IGI Global. doi:10.4018/978-1-5225-4769-3.ch012

Chakraborty, C., Gupta, B., & Ghosh, S. K. (2016). Mobile Telemedicine Systems for Remote Patient's Chronic Wound Monitoring. In A. Moumtzoglou (Ed.), *M-Health Innovations for Patient-Centered Care* (pp. 213–239). Hershey, PA: IGI Global. doi:10.4018/978-1-4666-9861-1.ch011

Chakraborty, S., Chatterjee, S., Ashour, A. S., Mali, K., & Dey, N. (2018). Intelligent Computing in Medical Imaging: A Study. In N. Dey (Ed.), *Advancements in Applied Metaheuristic Computing* (pp. 143–163). Hershey, PA: IGI Global. doi:10.4018/978-1-5225-4151-6.ch006

Chavez, A., & Kovarik, C. (2017). Open Source Technology for Medical Practice in Developing Countries. In K. Moahi, K. Bwalya, & P. Sebina (Eds.), *Health Information Systems and the Advancement of Medical Practice in Developing Countries* (pp. 33–59). Hershey, PA: IGI Global. doi:10.4018/978-1-5225-2262-1.ch003

Chen, E. T. (2016). Examining the Influence of Information Technology on Modern Health Care. In P. Manolitzas, E. Grigoroudis, N. Matsatsinis, & D. Yannacopoulos (Eds.), *Effective Methods for Modern Healthcare Service Quality and Evaluation* (pp. 110–136). Hershey, PA: IGI Global. doi:10.4018/978-1-4666-9961-8.ch006

Chin, S. (2016). Surviving Sandy: Recovering Collections after a Natural Disaster. In E. Decker & J. Townes (Eds.), *Handbook of Research on Disaster Management and Contingency Planning in Modern Libraries* (pp. 366–388). Hershey, PA: IGI Global. doi:10.4018/978-1-4666-8624-3.ch016

Chojnacki, M., & Wójcik, A. (2016). Security and the Role of New Technologies and Innovation in Medical Ethics. In A. Rosiek & K. Leksowski (Eds.), *Organizational Culture and Ethics in Modern Medicine* (pp. 52–77). Hershey, PA: IGI Global. doi:10.4018/978-1-4666-9658-7.ch003

Cılız, N., Yıldırım, H., & Temizel, Ş. (2016). Structure Development for Effective Medical Waste and Hazardous Waste Management System. In U. Akkucuk (Ed.), *Handbook of Research on Waste Management Techniques for Sustainability* (pp. 303–327). Hershey, PA: IGI Global. doi:10.4018/978-1-4666-9723-2.ch016

Ciufudean, C. (2018). Innovative Formalism for Biological Data Analysis. In M. Khosrow-Pour, D.B.A. (Ed.), Encyclopedia of Information Science and Technology, Fourth Edition (pp. 1814-1824). Hershey, PA: IGI Global. doi:10.4018/978-1-5225-2255-3.ch158

Ciufudean, C., & Ciufudean, O. (2016). Tele-Monitoring for Medical Diagnosis Availability. In M. Cruz-Cunha, I. Miranda, R. Martinho, & R. Rijo (Eds.), *Encyclopedia of E-Health and Telemedicine* (pp. 401–411). Hershey, PA: IGI Global. doi:10.4018/978-1-4666-9978-6.ch032

Colaguori, R., & Danesi, M. (2017). Medical Semiotics: A Revisitation and an Exhortation. *International Journal of Semiotics and Visual Rhetoric*, *1*(1), 11–18. doi:10.4018/IJSVR.2017010102

Cole, A. W., & Salek, T. A. (2017). Adopting a Parasocial Connection to Overcome Professional Kakoethos in Online Health Information. In M. Folk & S. Apostel (Eds.), *Establishing and Evaluating Digital Ethos and Online Credibility* (pp. 104–120). Hershey, PA: IGI Global. doi:10.4018/978-1-5225-1072-7.ch006

Contreras, E. C., & Puente, G. J. (2016). How to Identify Rheumatic Diseases by General Physicians. In T. Gasmelseid (Ed.), *Advancing Pharmaceutical Processes and Tools for Improved Health Outcomes* (pp. 136–166). Hershey, PA: IGI Global. doi:10.4018/978-1-5225-0248-7.ch006

D'Andrea, A., Ferri, F., & Grifoni, P. (2016). RFID Technologies in Healthcare Setting: Applications and Future Perspectives. *International Journal of Computers in Clinical Practice*, *1*(1), 15–27. doi:10.4018/IJCCP.2016010102

Damianakis, A., Kallonis, P., Loudos, G., Tsatsos, D., & Tsoukalis, A. (2016). Exploiting 3D Medical Equipment Simulations to Support Biomedical Engineering Academic Courses: Design Methodology and Implementation in a Small Scale National Project. In B. Khan (Ed.), *Revolutionizing Modern Education through Meaningful E-Learning Implementation* (pp. 277–295). Hershey, PA: IGI Global. doi:10.4018/978-1-5225-0466-5.ch015

Demiroz, E. (2016). Principles of Instructional Design for E-Learning and Online Learning Practices: Implications for Medical Education. In V. Wang (Ed.), *Handbook of Research on Advancing Health Education through Technology* (pp. 419–451). Hershey, PA: IGI Global. doi:10.4018/978-1-4666-9494-1.ch018

Deperlioglu, O. (2018). Intelligent Techniques Inspired by Nature and Used in Biomedical Engineering. In U. Kose, G. Guraksin, & O. Deperlioglu (Eds.), *Nature-Inspired Intelligent Techniques for Solving Biomedical Engineering Problems* (pp. 51–77). Hershey, PA: IGI Global. doi:10.4018/978-1-5225-4769-3.ch003

Dey, N., & Ashour, A. S. (2018). Meta-Heuristic Algorithms in Medical Image Segmentation: A Review. In N. Dey (Ed.), *Advancements in Applied Metaheuristic Computing* (pp. 185–203). Hershey, PA: IGI Global. doi:10.4018/978-1-5225-4151-6.ch008

Dey, N., Ashour, A. S., & Althoupety, A. S. (2017). Thermal Imaging in Medical Science. In V. Santhi (Ed.), *Recent Advances in Applied Thermal Imaging for Industrial Applications* (pp. 87–117). Hershey, PA: IGI Global. doi:10.4018/978-1-5225-2423-6.ch004

Di Virgilio, F., Camillo, A. A., & Camillo, I. C. (2017). The Impact of Social Network on Italian Users' Behavioural Intention for the Choice of a Medical Tourist Destination. *International Journal of Tourism and Hospitality Management in the Digital Age*, *1*(1), 36–49. doi:10.4018/IJTHMDA.2017010103

Dias, C. M., Ribeiro, A. G., & Furtado, S. F. (2016). An Overview about the Use of Healthcare Applications on Mobile Devices. In M. Cruz-Cunha, I. Miranda, R. Martinho, & R. Rijo (Eds.), *Encyclopedia of E-Health and Telemedicine* (pp. 285–298). Hershey, PA: IGI Global. doi:10.4018/978-1-4666-9978-6.ch024

Dogra, A. K., & Dogra, P. (2017). The Medical Tourism Industry in the BRIC Nations: An Indian Analysis. In M. Dhiman (Ed.), *Opportunities and Challenges for Tourism and Hospitality in the BRIC Nations* (pp. 320–336). Hershey, PA: IGI Global. doi:10.4018/978-1-5225-0708-6.ch020

Drowos, J. L., & Wood, S. K. (2017). Preparing Future Physicians to Adapt to the Changing Health Care System: Promoting Humanism through Curricular Design. In V. Bryan & J. Bird (Eds.), *Healthcare Community Synergism between Patients, Practitioners, and Researchers* (pp. 106–125). Hershey, PA: IGI Global. doi:10.4018/978-1-5225-0640-9.ch006

Dulam, K. (2017). Medical Patents and Impact on Availability and Affordability of Essential Medicines in India. In R. Aggarwal & R. Kaur (Eds.), *Patent Law and Intellectual Property in the Medical Field* (pp. 41–57). Hershey, PA: IGI Global. doi:10.4018/978-1-5225-2414-4.ch003

Dutta, P. (2017). Decision Making in Medical Diagnosis via Distance Measures on Interval Valued Fuzzy Sets. *International Journal of System Dynamics Applications*, *6*(4), 63–83. doi:10.4018/IJSDA.2017100104

Edoh, T. O., Pawar, P. A., Brügge, B., & Teege, G. (2016). A Multidisciplinary Remote Healthcare Delivery System to Increase Health Care Access, Pathology Screening, and Treatment in Developing Countries: The Case of Benin. *International Journal of Healthcare Information Systems and Informatics*, *11*(4), 1–31. doi:10.4018/IJHISI.2016100101

El Guemhioui, K., & Demurjian, S. A. (2017). Semantic Reconciliation of Electronic Health Records Using Semantic Web Technologies. *International Journal of Information Technology and Web Engineering*, *12*(2), 26–48. doi:10.4018/IJITWE.2017040102

Ellouze, N., Rekhis, S., & Boudriga, N. (2016). Forensic Investigation of Digital Crimes in Healthcare Applications. In O. Isafiade & A. Bagula (Eds.), *Data Mining Trends and Applications in Criminal Science and Investigations* (pp. 169–210). Hershey, PA: IGI Global. doi:10.4018/978-1-5225-0463-4.ch007

Eneanya, A. N. (2016). Health Policy Implementation and Its Barriers: The Case Study of US Health System. In R. Gholipour & K. Rouzbehani (Eds.), *Social, Economic, and Political Perspectives on Public Health Policy-Making* (pp. 42–63). Hershey, PA: IGI Global. doi:10.4018/978-1-4666-9944-1.ch003

Entico, G. J. (2016). Knowledge Management and the Medical Health Librarians: A Perception Study. In J. Yap, M. Perez, M. Ayson, & G. Entico (Eds.), *Special Library Administration, Standardization and Technological Integration* (pp. 52–77). Hershey, PA: IGI Global. doi:10.4018/978-1-4666-9542-9.ch003

Ferradji, M. A., & Zidani, A. (2016). Collaborative Environment for Remote Clinical Reasoning Learning. *International Journal of E-Health and Medical Communications*, *7*(4), 62–81. doi:10.4018/IJEHMC.2016100104

Fisher, J. (2018). Sociological Perspectives on Improving Medical Diagnosis Emphasizing CAD. In M. Khosrow-Pour, D.B.A. (Ed.), Encyclopedia of Information Science and Technology, Fourth Edition (pp. 1017-1024). Hershey, PA: IGI Global. doi:10.4018/978-1-5225-2255-3.ch088

Flores, C. D., Respício, A., Coelho, H., Bez, M. R., & Fonseca, J. M. (2016). Simulation for Medical Training. In M. Cruz-Cunha, I. Miranda, R. Martinho, & R. Rijo (Eds.), *Encyclopedia of E-Health and Telemedicine* (pp. 827–842). Hershey, PA: IGI Global. doi:10.4018/978-1-4666-9978-6.ch064

Frank, E. M. (2018). Healthcare Education: Integrating Simulation Technologies. In V. Bryan, A. Musgrove, & J. Powers (Eds.), *Handbook of Research on Human Development in the Digital Age* (pp. 163–182). Hershey, PA: IGI Global. doi:10.4018/978-1-5225-2838-8.ch008

Garner, G. (2018). Foundations for Yoga Practice in Rehabilitation. In S. Telles & N. Singh (Eds.), *Research-Based Perspectives on the Psychophysiology of Yoga* (pp. 263–307). Hershey, PA: IGI Global. doi:10.4018/978-1-5225-2788-6.ch015

Gasmelseid, T. M. (2016). Improving Pharmaceutical Care through the Use of Intelligent Pharmacoinformatics. In T. Gasmelseid (Ed.), *Advancing Pharmaceutical Processes and Tools for Improved Health Outcomes* (pp. 167–188). Hershey, PA: IGI Global. doi:10.4018/978-1-5225-0248-7.ch007

Gavurová, B., Kováč, V., & Šoltés, M. (2018). Medical Equipment and Economic Determinants of Its Structure and Regulation in the Slovak Republic. In M. Khosrow-Pour, D.B.A. (Ed.), Encyclopedia of Information Science and Technology, Fourth Edition (pp. 5841-5852). Hershey, PA: IGI Global. doi:10.4018/978-1-5225-2255-3.ch508

Ge, X., Wang, Q., Huang, K., Law, V., & Thomas, D. C. (2017). Designing Simulated Learning Environments and Facilitating Authentic Learning Experiences in Medical Education. In J. Stefaniak (Ed.), *Advancing Medical Education Through Strategic Instructional Design* (pp. 77–100). Hershey, PA: IGI Global. doi:10.4018/978-1-5225-2098-6.ch004

Gewald, H., & Gewald, C. (2018). Inhibitors of Physicians' Use of Mandatory Hospital Information Systems (HIS). *International Journal of Healthcare Information Systems and Informatics, 13*(1), 29–44. doi:10.4018/IJHISI.2018010103

Ghosh, D., & Dinda, S. (2017). Health Infrastructure and Economic Development in India. In R. Das (Ed.), *Social, Health, and Environmental Infrastructures for Economic Growth* (pp. 99–119). Hershey, PA: IGI Global. doi:10.4018/978-1-5225-2364-2.ch006

Ghosh, K., & Sen, K. C. (2017). The Potential of Crowdsourcing in the Health Care Industry. In N. Wickramasinghe (Ed.), *Handbook of Research on Healthcare Administration and Management* (pp. 418–427). Hershey, PA: IGI Global. doi:10.4018/978-1-5225-0920-2.ch024

Ghrab, S., & Saad, I. (2016). Identifying Crucial Know-How and Knowing-That for Medical Decision Support. *International Journal of Decision Support System Technology*, *8*(4), 14–33. doi:10.4018/IJDSST.2016100102

Giokas, K., Tsirmpas, C., Anastasiou, A., Iliopoulou, D., Costarides, V., & Koutsouris, D. (2016). Contemporary Heart Failure Treatment Based on Improved Knowledge and Personalized Care of Comorbidities. In D. Fotiadis (Ed.), *Handbook of Research on Trends in the Diagnosis and Treatment of Chronic Conditions* (pp. 301–314). Hershey, PA: IGI Global. doi:10.4018/978-1-4666-8828-5.ch014

Gopalan, V., Chan, E., & Ho, D. T. (2018). Deliberate Self-Harm and Suicide Ideology in Medical Students. In C. Smith (Ed.), *Exploring the Pressures of Medical Education From a Mental Health and Wellness Perspective* (pp. 122–143). Hershey, PA: IGI Global. doi:10.4018/978-1-5225-2811-1.ch005

Goswami, S., Dey, U., Roy, P., Ashour, A., & Dey, N. (2017). Medical Video Processing: Concept and Applications. In N. Dey, A. Ashour, & P. Patra (Eds.), *Feature Detectors and Motion Detection in Video Processing* (pp. 1–17). Hershey, PA: IGI Global. doi:10.4018/978-1-5225-1025-3.ch001

Goswami, S., Mahanta, K., Goswami, S., Jigdung, T., & Devi, T. P. (2018). Ageing and Cancer: The Epigenetic Basis, Alternative Treatment, and Care. In B. Prasad & S. Akbar (Eds.), *Handbook of Research on Geriatric Health, Treatment, and Care* (pp. 206–235). Hershey, PA: IGI Global. doi:10.4018/978-1-5225-3480-8.ch012

Gouva, M. I. (2017). The Psychological Impact of Medical Error on Patients, Family Members, and Health Professionals. In M. Riga (Ed.), *Impact of Medical Errors and Malpractice on Health Economics, Quality, and Patient Safety* (pp. 171–196). Hershey, PA: IGI Global. doi:10.4018/978-1-5225-2337-6.ch007

Gürcü, M., & Tengilimoğlu, D. (2017). Health Tourism-Based Destination Marketing. In A. Bayraktar & C. Uslay (Eds.), *Strategic Place Branding Methodologies and Theory for Tourist Attraction* (pp. 308–331). Hershey, PA: IGI Global. doi:10.4018/978-1-5225-0579-2.ch015

Gürsel, G. (2016). Mobility in Healthcare: M-Health. In A. Panagopoulos (Ed.), *Handbook of Research on Next Generation Mobile Communication Systems* (pp. 485–511). Hershey, PA: IGI Global. doi:10.4018/978-1-4666-8732-5.ch019

Gürsel, G. (2017). For Better Healthcare Mining Health Data. In S. Bhattacharyya, S. De, I. Pan, & P. Dutta (Eds.), *Intelligent Multidimensional Data Clustering and Analysis* (pp. 135–158). Hershey, PA: IGI Global. doi:10.4018/978-1-5225-1776-4.ch006

Guzman-Lugo, G., Lopez-Martinez, M., Lopez-Ramirez, B., & Avila-Vazquez, D. (2016). City-Driven Approach to Determine Health Services Based on Current User Location and Collaborative Information. *International Journal of Knowledge Society Research, 7*(1), 53–62. doi:10.4018/IJKSR.2016010104

Gyaase, P. O., Darko-Lartey, R., William, H., & Borkloe, F. (2017). Towards an Integrated Electronic Medical Records System for Quality Healthcare in Ghana: An Exploratory Factor Analysis. *International Journal of Computers in Clinical Practice, 2*(2), 38–55. doi:10.4018/IJCCP.2017070103

Handayani, P. W., Sandhyaduhita, P. I., Hidayanto, A. N., Pinem, A. A., Fajrina, H. R., Junus, K. M., ... Ayuningtyas, D. (2016). Integrated Hospital Information System Architecture Design in Indonesia. In T. Iyamu & A. Tatnall (Eds.), *Maximizing Healthcare Delivery and Management through Technology Integration* (pp. 207–236). Hershey, PA: IGI Global. doi:10.4018/978-1-4666-9446-0.ch013

Hanel, P. (2017). Is China Catching Up?: Health-Related Applications of Biotechnology. In T. Bas & J. Zhao (Eds.), *Comparative Approaches to Biotechnology Development and Use in Developed and Emerging Nations* (pp. 465–520). Hershey, PA: IGI Global. doi:10.4018/978-1-5225-1040-6.ch016

Harmsen, C. A., & Royle, R. N. (2016). St. Stephen's Hospital Hervey Bay: Study of Developing a Digital Hospital. In J. Moon & M. Galea (Eds.), *Improving Health Management through Clinical Decision Support Systems* (pp. 127–153). Hershey, PA: IGI Global. doi:10.4018/978-1-4666-9432-3.ch006

Harp, D., Shim, R. S., Johnson, J., Harp, J. A., Wilcox, W. C., & Wilcox, J. K. (2016). Race and Gender Inequalities in Medicine and Biomedical Research. In U. Thomas & J. Drake (Eds.), *Critical Research on Sexism and Racism in STEM Fields* (pp. 115–134). Hershey, PA: IGI Global. doi:10.4018/978-1-5225-0174-9.ch006

Hartman, A., & Brown, S. (2017). Synergism through Therapeutic Visual Arts. In V. Bryan & J. Bird (Eds.), *Healthcare Community Synergism between Patients, Practitioners, and Researchers* (pp. 29–48). Hershey, PA: IGI Global. doi:10.4018/978-1-5225-0640-9.ch002

Hazra, J., Chowdhury, A. R., & Dutta, P. (2016). Cluster Based Medical Image Registration Using Optimized Neural Network. In S. Bhattacharyya, P. Banerjee, D. Majumdar, & P. Dutta (Eds.), *Handbook of Research on Advanced Hybrid Intelligent Techniques and Applications* (pp. 551–581). Hershey, PA: IGI Global. doi:10.4018/978-1-4666-9474-3.ch018

Hung, S., Huang, W., Yen, D. C., Chang, S., & Lu, C. (2016). Effect of Information Service Competence and Contextual Factors on the Effectiveness of Strategic Information Systems Planning in Hospitals. *Journal of Global Information Management, 24*(1), 14–36. doi:10.4018/JGIM.2016010102

Iltchev, P., Śliwczyński, A., Szynkiewicz, P., & Marczak, M. (2016). Mobile Health Applications Assisting Patients with Chronic Diseases: Examples from Asthma Care. In A. Moumtzoglou (Ed.), *M-Health Innovations for Patient-Centered Care* (pp. 170–196). Hershey, PA: IGI Global. doi:10.4018/978-1-4666-9861-1.ch009

Iqbal, S., Ahmad, S., & Willis, I. (2017). Influencing Factors for Adopting Technology Enhanced Learning in the Medical Schools of Punjab, Pakistan. *International Journal of Information and Communication Technology Education, 13*(3), 27–39. doi:10.4018/IJICTE.2017070103

Jagan, J., Dalkiliç, Y., & Samui, P. (2016). Utilization of SVM, LSSVM and GP for Predicting the Medical Waste Generation. In G. Hua (Ed.), *Smart Cities as a Solution for Reducing Urban Waste and Pollution* (pp. 224–251). Hershey, PA: IGI Global. doi:10.4018/978-1-5225-0302-6.ch008

Jagiello, K., Sosnowska, A., Mikolajczyk, A., & Puzyn, T. (2017). Nanomaterials in Medical Devices: Regulations' Review and Future Perspectives. *Journal of Nanotoxicology and Nanomedicine, 2*(2), 1–11. doi:10.4018/JNN.2017070101

Jena, T. K. (2018). Skill Training Process in Medicine Through Distance Mode. In U. Pandey & V. Indrakanti (Eds.), *Optimizing Open and Distance Learning in Higher Education Institutions* (pp. 228–243). Hershey, PA: IGI Global. doi:10.4018/978-1-5225-2624-7.ch010

Jesus, Â., & Gomes, M. J. (2016). Web 2.0 Tools in Biomedical and Pharmaceutical Education: Updated Review and Commentary. In T. Gasmelseid (Ed.), *Advancing Pharmaceutical Processes and Tools for Improved Health Outcomes* (pp. 52–78). Hershey, PA: IGI Global. doi:10.4018/978-1-5225-0248-7.ch003

Joseph, V., & Miller, J. M. (2018). Medical Students' Perceived Stigma in Seeking Care: A Cultural Perspective. In C. Smith (Ed.), *Exploring the Pressures of Medical Education From a Mental Health and Wellness Perspective* (pp. 44–67). Hershey, PA: IGI Global. doi:10.4018/978-1-5225-2811-1.ch002

Joyce, B. L., & Swanberg, S. M. (2017). Using Backward Design for Competency-Based Undergraduate Medical Education. In J. Stefaniak (Ed.), *Advancing Medical Education Through Strategic Instructional Design* (pp. 53–76). Hershey, PA: IGI Global. doi:10.4018/978-1-5225-2098-6.ch003

Kaljo, K., & Jacques, L. (2018). Flipping the Medical School Classroom. In M. Khosrow-Pour, D.B.A. (Ed.), Encyclopedia of Information Science and Technology, Fourth Edition (pp. 5800-5809). Hershey, PA: IGI Global. doi:10.4018/978-1-5225-2255-3.ch504

Karon, R. (2016). Utilisation of Health Information Systems for Service Delivery in the Namibian Environment. In T. Iyamu & A. Tatnall (Eds.), *Maximizing Healthcare Delivery and Management through Technology Integration* (pp. 169–183). Hershey, PA: IGI Global. doi:10.4018/978-1-4666-9446-0.ch011

Kasina, H., Bahubalendruni, M. V., & Botcha, R. (2017). Robots in Medicine: Past, Present and Future. *International Journal of Manufacturing, Materials, and Mechanical Engineering*, *7*(4), 44–64. doi:10.4018/IJMMME.2017100104

Katehakis, D. G. (2018). Electronic Medical Record Implementation Challenges for the National Health System in Greece. *International Journal of Reliable and Quality E-Healthcare*, *7*(1), 16–30. doi:10.4018/IJRQEH.2018010102

Katz, A., & Shtub, A. (2016). Design and Build a Wizard of Oz (WOZ) Telemedicine Simulator Platform. In M. Cruz-Cunha, I. Miranda, R. Martinho, & R. Rijo (Eds.), *Encyclopedia of E-Health and Telemedicine* (pp. 128–141). Hershey, PA: IGI Global. doi:10.4018/978-1-4666-9978-6.ch011

Kaur, P. D., & Sharma, P. (2017). Success Dimensions of ICTs in Healthcare. In B. Singh (Ed.), *Computational Tools and Techniques for Biomedical Signal Processing* (pp. 149–173). Hershey, PA: IGI Global. doi:10.4018/978-1-5225-0660-7.ch007

Kaushik, P. (2018). Comorbidity of Medical and Psychiatric Disorders in Geriatric Population: Treatment and Care. In B. Prasad & S. Akbar (Eds.), *Handbook of Research on Geriatric Health, Treatment, and Care* (pp. 448–474). Hershey, PA: IGI Global. doi:10.4018/978-1-5225-3480-8.ch025

Khachane, M. Y. (2017). Organ-Based Medical Image Classification Using Support Vector Machine. *International Journal of Synthetic Emotions*, *8*(1), 18–30. doi:10.4018/IJSE.2017010102

Kirci, P. (2018). Intelligent Techniques for Analysis of Big Data About Healthcare and Medical Records. In N. Shah & M. Mittal (Eds.), *Handbook of Research on Promoting Business Process Improvement Through Inventory Control Techniques* (pp. 559–582). Hershey, PA: IGI Global. doi:10.4018/978-1-5225-3232-3.ch029

Kldiashvili, E. (2016). Cloud Computing as the Useful Resource for Application of the Medical Information System for Quality Assurance Purposes. *International Journal of Computers in Clinical Practice*, *1*(2), 1–23. doi:10.4018/IJCCP.2016070101

Kldiashvili, E. (2018). Cloud Approach for the Medical Information System: MIS on Cloud. In M. Khosrow-Pour (Ed.), *Incorporating Nature-Inspired Paradigms in Computational Applications* (pp. 238–261). Hershey, PA: IGI Global. doi:10.4018/978-1-5225-5020-4.ch008

Kldiashvili, E., Burduli, A., Ghortlishvili, G., & Sheklashvili, I. (2016). Georgian Experience in Telecytology. In M. Cruz-Cunha, I. Miranda, R. Martinho, & R. Rijo (Eds.), *Encyclopedia of E-Health and Telemedicine* (pp. 62–71). Hershey, PA: IGI Global. doi:10.4018/978-1-4666-9978-6.ch006

Ko, H., Mesicek, L., Choi, J., Choi, J., & Hwang, S. (2018). A Study on Secure Contents Strategies for Applications With DRM on Cloud Computing. *International Journal of Cloud Applications and Computing*, *8*(1), 143–153. doi:10.4018/IJCAC.2018010107

Komendziński, T., Dreszer-Drogorób, J., Mikołajewska, E., Mikołajewski, D., & Bałaj, B. (2016). Interdisciplinary Education for Research and Everyday Clinical Practice: Lessons Learned from InteRDoCTor Project. In A. Rosiek & K. Leksowski (Eds.), *Organizational Culture and Ethics in Modern Medicine* (pp. 78–110). Hershey, PA: IGI Global. doi:10.4018/978-1-4666-9658-7.ch004

Komendziński, T., Mikołajewska, E., & Mikołajewski, D. (2018). Cross-Cultural Decision-Making in Healthcare: Theory and Practical Application in Real Clinical Conditions. In A. Rosiek-Kryszewska & K. Leksowski (Eds.), *Healthcare Administration for Patient Safety and Engagement* (pp. 276–298). Hershey, PA: IGI Global. doi:10.4018/978-1-5225-3946-9.ch015

Konecny, L. T. (2018). Medical School Wellness Initiatives. In C. Smith (Ed.), *Exploring the Pressures of Medical Education From a Mental Health and Wellness Perspective* (pp. 209–228). Hershey, PA: IGI Global. doi:10.4018/978-1-5225-2811-1.ch009

Konieczna, A., & Słomkowski, P. (2016). Confrontation of Human Rights in Daily Clinical Situations. In A. Rosiek & K. Leksowski (Eds.), *Organizational Culture and Ethics in Modern Medicine* (pp. 255–281). Hershey, PA: IGI Global. doi:10.4018/978-1-4666-9658-7.ch011

Kromrei, H., Solomonson, W. L., & Juzych, M. S. (2017). Teaching Residents How to Teach. In J. Stefaniak (Ed.), *Advancing Medical Education Through Strategic Instructional Design* (pp. 164–185). Hershey, PA: IGI Global. doi:10.4018/978-1-5225-2098-6.ch008

Kulkarni, S., Savyanavar, A., Kulkarni, P., Stranieri, A., & Ghorpade, V. (2018). Framework for Integration of Medical Image and Text-Based Report Retrieval to Support Radiological Diagnosis. In M. Kolekar & V. Kumar (Eds.), *Biomedical Signal and Image Processing in Patient Care* (pp. 86–122). Hershey, PA: IGI Global. doi:10.4018/978-1-5225-2829-6.ch006

Kumar, A., & Sarkar, B. K. (2018). Performance Analysis of Nature-Inspired Algorithms-Based Bayesian Prediction Models for Medical Data Sets. In U. Singh, A. Tiwari, & R. Singh (Eds.), *Soft-Computing-Based Nonlinear Control Systems Design* (pp. 134–155). Hershey, PA: IGI Global. doi:10.4018/978-1-5225-3531-7.ch007

Kurtz, R. S. (2016). Fortitude: A Study of African Americans in Surgery in New York City. In U. Thomas & J. Drake (Eds.), *Critical Research on Sexism and Racism in STEM Fields* (pp. 153–169). Hershey, PA: IGI Global. doi:10.4018/978-1-5225-0174-9.ch009

Labbadi, W., & Akaichi, J. (2017). Efficient Algorithm for Answering Fuzzy Medical Requests in Pervasive Healthcare Information Systems. *International Journal of Healthcare Information Systems and Informatics*, *12*(2), 46–64. doi:10.4018/IJHISI.2017040103

Lagumdzija, A., & Swing, V. K. (2017). Health, Digitalization, and Individual Empowerment. In F. Topor (Ed.), *Handbook of Research on Individualism and Identity in the Globalized Digital Age* (pp. 380–402). Hershey, PA: IGI Global. doi:10.4018/978-1-5225-0522-8.ch017

Lamey, T. W., & Davidson-Shivers, G. V. (2017). Instructional Strategies and Sequencing. In J. Stefaniak (Ed.), *Advancing Medical Education Through Strategic Instructional Design* (pp. 30–52). Hershey, PA: IGI Global. doi:10.4018/978-1-5225-2098-6.ch002

Leon, G. (2017). The Role of Forensic Medicine in Medical Errors. In M. Riga (Ed.), *Impact of Medical Errors and Malpractice on Health Economics, Quality, and Patient Safety* (pp. 144–170). Hershey, PA: IGI Global. doi:10.4018/978-1-5225-2337-6.ch006

Lidia, B., Federica, G., & Maria, V. E. (2016). The Patient-Centered Medicine as the Theoretical Framework for Patient Engagement. In G. Graffigna (Ed.), *Promoting Patient Engagement and Participation for Effective Healthcare Reform* (pp. 25–39). Hershey, PA: IGI Global. doi:10.4018/978-1-4666-9992-2.ch002

Love, L., & McDowelle, D. (2018). Developing a Comprehensive Wellness Program for Medical Students. In C. Smith (Ed.), *Exploring the Pressures of Medical Education From a Mental Health and Wellness Perspective* (pp. 190–208). Hershey, PA: IGI Global. doi:10.4018/978-1-5225-2811-1.ch008

Lovell, K. L. (2017). Development and Evaluation of Neuroscience Computer-Based Modules for Medical Students: Instructional Design Principles and Effectiveness. In J. Stefaniak (Ed.), *Advancing Medical Education Through Strategic Instructional Design* (pp. 262–276). Hershey, PA: IGI Global. doi:10.4018/978-1-5225-2098-6.ch013

Lubin, R., & Hamlin, M. D. (2018). Medical Student Burnout: A Social Cognitive Learning Perspective on Medical Student Mental Health and Wellness. In C. Smith (Ed.), *Exploring the Pressures of Medical Education From a Mental Health and Wellness Perspective* (pp. 92–121). Hershey, PA: IGI Global. doi:10.4018/978-1-5225-2811-1.ch004

Luk, C. Y. (2018). Moving Towards Universal Health Coverage: Challenges for the Present and Future in China. In B. Fong, A. Ng, & P. Yuen (Eds.), *Sustainable Health and Long-Term Care Solutions for an Aging Population* (pp. 19–45). Hershey, PA: IGI Global. doi:10.4018/978-1-5225-2633-9.ch002

Mahat, M., & Pettigrew, A. (2017). The Regulatory Environment of Non-Profit Higher Education and Research Institutions and Its Implications for Managerial Strategy: The Case of Medical Education and Research. In L. West & A. Worthington (Eds.), *Handbook of Research on Emerging Business Models and Managerial Strategies in the Nonprofit Sector* (pp. 336–351). Hershey, PA: IGI Global. doi:10.4018/978-1-5225-2537-0.ch017

Maitra, I. K., & Bandhyopadhyaay, S. K. (2017). Adaptive Edge Detection Method towards Features Extraction from Diverse Medical Imaging Technologies. In S. Bhattacharyya, S. De, I. Pan, & P. Dutta (Eds.), *Intelligent Multidimensional Data Clustering and Analysis* (pp. 159–192). Hershey, PA: IGI Global. doi:10.4018/978-1-5225-1776-4.ch007

Mangu, V. P. (2017). Mobile Health Care: A Technology View. In C. Bhatt & S. Peddoju (Eds.), *Cloud Computing Systems and Applications in Healthcare* (pp. 1–18). Hershey, PA: IGI Global. doi:10.4018/978-1-5225-1002-4.ch001

Manirabona, A., Fourati, L. C., & Boudjit, S. (2017). Investigation on Healthcare Monitoring Systems: Innovative Services and Applications. *International Journal of E-Health and Medical Communications*, *8*(1), 1–18. doi:10.4018/IJEHMC.2017010101

Mannai, M. M., & Karâa, W. B. (2016). Biomedical Image Processing Overview. In W. Karâa & N. Dey (Eds.), *Biomedical Image Analysis and Mining Techniques for Improved Health Outcomes* (pp. 1–12). Hershey, PA: IGI Global. doi:10.4018/978-1-4666-8811-7.ch001

Manzoor, A. (2016). RFID in Health Care-Building Smart Hospitals for Quality Healthcare. *International Journal of User-Driven Healthcare, 6*(2), 21–45. doi:10.4018/IJUDH.2016070102

Marwan, M., Kartit, A., & Ouahmane, H. (2018). A Framework to Secure Medical Image Storage in Cloud Computing Environment. *Journal of Electronic Commerce in Organizations, 16*(1), 1–16. doi:10.4018/JECO.2018010101

Masoud, M. P., Nejad, M. K., Darebaghi, H., Chavoshi, M., & Farahani, M. (2018). The Decision Support System and Conventional Method of Telephone Triage by Nurses in Emergency Medical Services: A Comparative Investigation. *International Journal of E-Business Research, 14*(1), 77–88. doi:10.4018/IJEBR.2018010105

McDonald, W. G., Martin, M., & Salzberg, L. D. (2018). From Medical Student to Medical Resident: Graduate Medical Education and Mental Health in the United States. In C. Smith (Ed.), *Exploring the Pressures of Medical Education From a Mental Health and Wellness Perspective* (pp. 145–169). Hershey, PA: IGI Global. doi:10.4018/978-1-5225-2811-1.ch006

Medhekar, A. (2017). The Role of Social Media for Knowledge Dissemination in Medical Tourism: A Case of India. In R. Chugh (Ed.), *Harnessing Social Media as a Knowledge Management Tool* (pp. 25–54). Hershey, PA: IGI Global. doi:10.4018/978-1-5225-0495-5.ch002

Medhekar, A., & Haq, F. (2018). Urbanization and New Jobs Creation in Healthcare Services in India: Challenges and Opportunities. In U. Benna & I. Benna (Eds.), *Urbanization and Its Impact on Socio-Economic Growth in Developing Regions* (pp. 198–218). Hershey, PA: IGI Global. doi:10.4018/978-1-5225-2659-9.ch010

Mehta, G., Dutta, M. K., & Kim, P. S. (2016). An Efficient and Lossless Cryptosystem for Security in Tele-Ophthalmology Applications Using Chaotic Theory. *International Journal of E-Health and Medical Communications, 7*(4), 28–47. doi:10.4018/IJEHMC.2016100102

Mehta, P. (2017). Framework of Indian Healthcare System and its Challenges: An Insight. In V. Bryan & J. Bird (Eds.), *Healthcare Community Synergism between Patients, Practitioners, and Researchers* (pp. 247–271). Hershey, PA: IGI Global. doi:10.4018/978-1-5225-0640-9.ch011

Metelmann, B., & Metelmann, C. (2016). M-Health in Prehospital Emergency Medicine: Experiences from the EU funded Project LiveCity. In A. Moumtzoglou (Ed.), *M-Health Innovations for Patient-Centered Care* (pp. 197–212). Hershey, PA: IGI Global. doi:10.4018/978-1-4666-9861-1.ch010

Mi, M. (2017). Informal Learning in Medical Education. In J. Stefaniak (Ed.), *Advancing Medical Education Through Strategic Instructional Design* (pp. 225–244). Hershey, PA: IGI Global. doi:10.4018/978-1-5225-2098-6.ch011

Miglioretti, M., Mariani, F., & Vecchio, L. (2016). Could Patient Engagement Promote a Health System Free From Malpractice Litigation Risk? In G. Graffigna (Ed.), *Promoting Patient Engagement and Participation for Effective Healthcare Reform* (pp. 240–264). Hershey, PA: IGI Global. doi:10.4018/978-1-4666-9992-2.ch012

Misra, S. C., & Bisui, S. (2016). Feasibility of Large Scale Implementation of Personalized Medicine in the Current Scenario. *International Journal of E-Health and Medical Communications*, *7*(2), 30–49. doi:10.4018/IJEHMC.2016040103

Misra, S. C., Bisui, S., & Fantazy, K. (2016). Identifying Critical Changes in Adoption of Personalized Medicine (PM) in Healthcare Management. *International Journal of E-Health and Medical Communications*, *7*(3), 1–15. doi:10.4018/IJEHMC.2016070101

Mohammadian, M., Hatzinakos, D., Spachos, P., & Jentzsh, R. (2016). An Intelligent and Secure Framework for Wireless Information Technology in Healthcare for User and Data Classification in Hospitals. In V. Wang (Ed.), *Handbook of Research on Advancing Health Education through Technology* (pp. 452–479). Hershey, PA: IGI Global. doi:10.4018/978-1-4666-9494-1.ch019

Mokeddem, S., & Atmani, B. (2016). Assessment of Clinical Decision Support Systems for Predicting Coronary Heart Disease. *International Journal of Operations Research and Information Systems*, *7*(3), 57–73. doi:10.4018/IJORIS.2016070104

Mokrzycka, A., & Kowalska-Bobko, I. (2016). Public Health Legislation and Patient's Rights: Health2020 Strategy, European Perspective. In A. Rosiek & K. Leksowski (Eds.), *Organizational Culture and Ethics in Modern Medicine* (pp. 298–322). Hershey, PA: IGI Global. doi:10.4018/978-1-4666-9658-7.ch013

Moon, J. D., & Galea, M. P. (2016). Overview of Clinical Decision Support Systems in Healthcare. In J. Moon & M. Galea (Eds.), *Improving Health Management through Clinical Decision Support Systems* (pp. 1–27). Hershey, PA: IGI Global. doi:10.4018/978-1-4666-9432-3.ch001

Mosadeghrad, A. M., & Woldemichael, A. (2017). Application of Quality Management in Promoting Patient Safety and Preventing Medical Errors. In M. Riga (Ed.), *Impact of Medical Errors and Malpractice on Health Economics, Quality, and Patient Safety* (pp. 91–112). Hershey, PA: IGI Global. doi:10.4018/978-1-5225-2337-6.ch004

Moumtzoglou, A. (2017). Digital Medicine: The Quality Standpoint. In A. Moumtzoglou (Ed.), *Design, Development, and Integration of Reliable Electronic Healthcare Platforms* (pp. 179–195). Hershey, PA: IGI Global. doi:10.4018/978-1-5225-1724-5.ch011

Moumtzoglou, A., & Pouliakis, A. (2018). Population Health Management and the Science of Individuality. *International Journal of Reliable and Quality E-Healthcare*, *7*(2), 1–26. doi:10.4018/IJRQEH.2018040101

Mpofu, C. (2016). International Medical Experiences Outbound New Zealand: An Economic and Medical Workforce Strategy. In D. Velliaris & D. Coleman-George (Eds.), *Handbook of Research on Study Abroad Programs and Outbound Mobility* (pp. 446–469). Hershey, PA: IGI Global. doi:10.4018/978-1-5225-0169-5.ch018

Mukhtar, W. F., & Abuelyaman, E. S. (2017). Opportunities and Challenges of Big Data in Healthcare. In N. Wickramasinghe (Ed.), *Handbook of Research on Healthcare Administration and Management* (pp. 47–58). Hershey, PA: IGI Global. doi:10.4018/978-1-5225-0920-2.ch004

Munugala, S., Brar, G. K., Syed, A., Mohammad, A., & Halgamuge, M. N. (2018). The Much Needed Security and Data Reforms of Cloud Computing in Medical Data Storage. In M. Lytras & P. Papadopoulou (Eds.), *Applying Big Data Analytics in Bioinformatics and Medicine* (pp. 99–113). Hershey, PA: IGI Global. doi:10.4018/978-1-5225-2607-0.ch005

Narasimhamurthy, A. (2016). An Overview of Machine Learning in Medical Image Analysis: Trends in Health Informatics. In N. Dey & A. Ashour (Eds.), *Classification and Clustering in Biomedical Signal Processing* (pp. 23–45). Hershey, PA: IGI Global. doi:10.4018/978-1-5225-0140-4.ch002

Ngara, R. (2017). Multiple Voices, Multiple Paths: Towards Dialogue between Western and Indigenous Medical Knowledge Systems. In P. Ngulube (Ed.), *Handbook of Research on Theoretical Perspectives on Indigenous Knowledge Systems in Developing Countries* (pp. 332–358). Hershey, PA: IGI Global. doi:10.4018/978-1-5225-0833-5.ch015

O'Connor, Y., & Heavin, C. (2018). Defining and Characterising the Landscape of eHealth. In M. Khosrow-Pour, D.B.A. (Ed.), Encyclopedia of Information Science and Technology, Fourth Edition (pp. 5864-5875). Hershey, PA: IGI Global. doi:10.4018/978-1-5225-2255-3.ch510

Ochonogor, W. C., & Okite-Amughoro, F. A. (2018). Building an Effective Digital Library in a University Teaching Hospital (UTH) in Nigeria. In A. Tella & T. Kwanya (Eds.), *Handbook of Research on Managing Intellectual Property in Digital Libraries* (pp. 184–204). Hershey, PA: IGI Global. doi:10.4018/978-1-5225-3093-0.ch010

Olaniran, B. A. (2016). ICTs, E-health, and Multidisciplinary Healthcare Teams: Promises and Challenges. *International Journal of Privacy and Health Information Management*, *4*(2), 62–75. doi:10.4018/IJPHIM.2016070105

Olaniran, B. A. (2016). ICT Use and Multidisciplinary Healthcare Teams in the Age of e-Health. *International Journal of Reliable and Quality E-Healthcare*, *5*(1), 18–31. doi:10.4018/IJRQEH.2016010102

Olivares, S. L., Cruz, A. G., Cabrera, M. V., Regalado, A. I., & García, J. E. (2017). An Assessment Study of Quality Model for Medical Schools in Mexico. In S. Mukerji & P. Tripathi (Eds.), *Handbook of Research on Administration, Policy, and Leadership in Higher Education* (pp. 404–439). Hershey, PA: IGI Global. doi:10.4018/978-1-5225-0672-0.ch016

Omidoyin, E. O., Opeke, R. O., & Osagbemi, G. K. (2016). Utilization Pattern and Privacy Issues in the use of Health Records for Research Practice by Doctors: Selected Nigerian Teaching Hospitals as Case Study. *International Journal of Privacy and Health Information Management*, *4*(1), 1–11. doi:10.4018/IJPHIM.2016010101

Omoruyi, E. A., & Omidele, F. (2018). Resident Physician and Medical Academic Faculty Burnout: A Review of Current Literature. In C. Smith (Ed.), *Exploring the Pressures of Medical Education From a Mental Health and Wellness Perspective* (pp. 171–189). Hershey, PA: IGI Global. doi:10.4018/978-1-5225-2811-1.ch007

Osop, H., & Sahama, T. (2016). Data-Driven and Practice-Based Evidence: Design and Development of Efficient and Effective Clinical Decision Support System. In J. Moon & M. Galea (Eds.), *Improving Health Management through Clinical Decision Support Systems* (pp. 295–328). Hershey, PA: IGI Global. doi:10.4018/978-1-4666-9432-3.ch014

Ossowski, R., & Izdebski, P. (2016). Ethical Aspects of Talking to a Patient. In A. Rosiek & K. Leksowski (Eds.), *Organizational Culture and Ethics in Modern Medicine* (pp. 203–235). Hershey, PA: IGI Global. doi:10.4018/978-1-4666-9658-7.ch009

Pandian, P. S. (2016). An Overview of Telemedicine Technologies for Healthcare Applications. *International Journal of Biomedical and Clinical Engineering*, *5*(2), 29–52. doi:10.4018/IJBCE.2016070103

Papadopoulou, P., Lytras, M., & Marouli, C. (2018). Bioinformatics as Applied to Medicine: Challenges Faced Moving from Big Data to Smart Data to Wise Data. In M. Lytras & P. Papadopoulou (Eds.), *Applying Big Data Analytics in Bioinformatics and Medicine* (pp. 1–25). Hershey, PA: IGI Global. doi:10.4018/978-1-5225-2607-0.ch001

Paraskou, A., & George, B. P. (2018). An Overview of Reproductive Tourism. In *Legal and Economic Considerations Surrounding Reproductive Tourism: Emerging Research and Opportunities* (pp. 1–17). Hershey, PA: IGI Global. doi:10.4018/978-1-5225-2694-0.ch001

Park, S., & Moon, J. (2016). Strategic Approach towards Clinical Information Security. In J. Moon & M. Galea (Eds.), *Improving Health Management through Clinical Decision Support Systems* (pp. 329–359). Hershey, PA: IGI Global. doi:10.4018/978-1-4666-9432-3.ch015

Pereira, D., Castro, A., Gomes, P., Areias, J. C., Reis, Z. S., Coimbra, M. T., & Cruz-Correia, R. (2016). Digital Auscultation: Challenges and Perspectives. In M. Cruz-Cunha, I. Miranda, R. Martinho, & R. Rijo (Eds.), *Encyclopedia of E-Health and Telemedicine* (pp. 910–927). Hershey, PA: IGI Global. doi:10.4018/978-1-4666-9978-6.ch070

Peters, R. A., & Cruz, M. (2016). The States as Generators of Incremental Change in American Health Care Policy: 1935 to 1965. In R. Gholipour & K. Rouzbehani (Eds.), *Social, Economic, and Political Perspectives on Public Health Policy-Making* (pp. 86–114). Hershey, PA: IGI Global. doi:10.4018/978-1-4666-9944-1.ch005

Phuritsabam, B., & Devi, A. B. (2017). Information Seeking Behavior of Medical Scientists at Jawaharlal Nehru Institute of Medical Science: A Study. In S. Ram (Ed.), *Library and Information Services for Bioinformatics Education and Research* (pp. 177–187). Hershey, PA: IGI Global. doi:10.4018/978-1-5225-1871-6.ch010

Pieczka, B. (2018). Management of Risk and Adverse Events in Medical Entities. In A. Rosiek-Kryszewska & K. Leksowski (Eds.), *Healthcare Administration for Patient Safety and Engagement* (pp. 31–46). Hershey, PA: IGI Global. doi:10.4018/978-1-5225-3946-9.ch003

Poduval, J. (2016). Curriculum Development. In *Optimizing Medicine Residency Training Programs* (pp. 45–102). Hershey, PA: IGI Global. doi:10.4018/978-1-4666-9527-6.ch003

Poduval, J. (2016). Ethics and Professionalism. In *Optimizing Medicine Residency Training Programs* (pp. 103–133). Hershey, PA: IGI Global. doi:10.4018/978-1-4666-9527-6.ch004

Poduval, J. (2016). Management Skills and Leadership. In *Optimizing Medicine Residency Training Programs* (pp. 182–205). Hershey, PA: IGI Global. doi:10.4018/978-1-4666-9527-6.ch008

Poduval, J. (2016). Medicine Residency Training. In *Optimizing Medicine Residency Training Programs* (pp. 1–27). Hershey, PA: IGI Global. doi:10.4018/978-1-4666-9527-6.ch001

Poduval, J. (2016). Personal Issues. In *Optimizing Medicine Residency Training Programs* (pp. 206–221). Hershey, PA: IGI Global. doi:10.4018/978-1-4666-9527-6.ch009

Poduval, J. (2017). Medical Errors: Impact on Health Care Quality. In M. Riga (Ed.), *Impact of Medical Errors and Malpractice on Health Economics, Quality, and Patient Safety* (pp. 33–60). Hershey, PA: IGI Global. doi:10.4018/978-1-5225-2337-6.ch002

Politis, D., Stagiopoulos, P., Aidona, S., Kyriafinis, G., & Constantinidis, I. (2018). Autonomous Learning and Skill Accreditation: A Paradigm for Medical Studies. In A. Kumar (Ed.), *Optimizing Student Engagement in Online Learning Environments* (pp. 266–296). Hershey, PA: IGI Global. doi:10.4018/978-1-5225-3634-5.ch012

Pomares-Quimbaya, A., Gonzalez, R. A., Quintero, S., Muñoz, O. M., Bohórquez, W. R., García, O. M., & Londoño, D. (2016). A Review of Existing Applications and Techniques for Narrative Text Analysis in Electronic Medical Records. In M. Cruz-Cunha, I. Miranda, R. Martinho, & R. Rijo (Eds.), *Encyclopedia of E-Health and Telemedicine* (pp. 796–811). Hershey, PA: IGI Global. doi:10.4018/978-1-4666-9978-6.ch062

Pomares-Quimbaya, A., González, R. A., Sierra, A., Daza, J. C., Muñoz, O., García, A., ... Bohórquez, W. R. (2017). ICT for Enabling the Quality Evaluation of Health Care Services: A Case Study in a General Hospital. In A. Moumtzoglou (Ed.), *Design, Development, and Integration of Reliable Electronic Healthcare Platforms* (pp. 196–210). Hershey, PA: IGI Global. doi:10.4018/978-1-5225-1724-5.ch012

Pouliakis, A., Margari, N., Karakitsou, E., Archondakis, S., & Karakitsos, P. (2018). Emerging Technologies Serving Cytopathology: Big Data, the Cloud, and Mobile Computing. In I. El Naqa (Ed.), *Emerging Developments and Practices in Oncology* (pp. 114–152). Hershey, PA: IGI Global. doi:10.4018/978-1-5225-3085-5.ch005

Queirós, A., Silva, A. G., Ferreira, A., Caravau, H., Cerqueira, M., & Rocha, N. P. (2016). Assessing Mobile Applications Considered Medical Devices. In M. Cruz-Cunha, I. Miranda, R. Martinho, & R. Rijo (Eds.), *Encyclopedia of E-Health and Telemedicine* (pp. 111–127). Hershey, PA: IGI Global. doi:10.4018/978-1-4666-9978-6.ch010

Raffaeli, L., Spinsante, S., & Gambi, E. (2016). Integrated Smart TV-Based Personal e-Health System. *International Journal of E-Health and Medical Communications*, *7*(1), 48–64. doi:10.4018/IJEHMC.2016010103

Rai, A., Kothari, R., & Singh, D. P. (2017). Assessment of Available Technologies for Hospital Waste Management: A Need for Society. In R. Singh, A. Singh, & V. Srivastava (Eds.), *Environmental Issues Surrounding Human Overpopulation* (pp. 172–188). Hershey, PA: IGI Global. doi:10.4018/978-1-5225-1683-5.ch010

Ramamoorthy, S., & Sivasubramaniam, R. (2018). Image Processing Including Medical Liver Imaging: Medical Image Processing from Big Data Perspective, Ultrasound Liver Images, Challenges. In M. Lytras & P. Papadopoulou (Eds.), *Applying Big Data Analytics in Bioinformatics and Medicine* (pp. 380–392). Hershey, PA: IGI Global. doi:10.4018/978-1-5225-2607-0.ch016

Rathor, G. P., & Gupta, S. K. (2017). Improving Multimodality Image Fusion through Integrate AFL and Wavelet Transform. In V. Tiwari, B. Tiwari, R. Thakur, & S. Gupta (Eds.), *Pattern and Data Analysis in Healthcare Settings* (pp. 143–157). Hershey, PA: IGI Global. doi:10.4018/978-1-5225-0536-5.ch008

Rawat, D. B., & Bhattacharya, S. (2016). Wireless Body Area Network for Healthcare Applications. In N. Meghanathan (Ed.), *Advanced Methods for Complex Network Analysis* (pp. 343–358). Hershey, PA: IGI Global. doi:10.4018/978-1-4666-9964-9.ch014

Rea, P. M. (2016). Advances in Anatomical and Medical Visualisation. In M. Pinheiro & D. Simões (Eds.), *Handbook of Research on Engaging Digital Natives in Higher Education Settings* (pp. 244–264). Hershey, PA: IGI Global. doi:10.4018/978-1-5225-0039-1.ch011

Rexhepi, H., & Persson, A. (2017). Challenges to Implementing IT Support for Evidence Based Practice Among Nurses and Assistant Nurses: A Qualitative Study. *Journal of Electronic Commerce in Organizations*, *15*(2), 61–76. doi:10.4018/JECO.2017040105

Reychav, I., & Azuri, J. (2016). Including Elderly Patients in Decision Making via Electronic Health Literacy. In M. Cruz-Cunha, I. Miranda, R. Martinho, & R. Rijo (Eds.), *Encyclopedia of E-Health and Telemedicine* (pp. 241–249). Hershey, PA: IGI Global. doi:10.4018/978-1-4666-9978-6.ch020

Richards, D., & Caldwell, P. H. (2016). Gamification to Improve Adherence to Clinical Treatment Advice: Improving Adherence to Clinical Treatment. In D. Novák, B. Tulu, & H. Brendryen (Eds.), *Handbook of Research on Holistic Perspectives in Gamification for Clinical Practice* (pp. 47–77). Hershey, PA: IGI Global. doi:10.4018/978-1-4666-9522-1.ch004

Rissman, B. (2016). Medical Conditions Associated with NLD. In B. Rissman (Ed.), *Medical and Educational Perspectives on Nonverbal Learning Disability in Children and Young Adults* (pp. 27–66). Hershey, PA: IGI Global. doi:10.4018/978-1-4666-9539-9.ch002

Rosiek, A. (2018). The Assessment of Actions of the Environment and the Impact of Preventive Medicine for Public Health in Poland. In A. Rosiek-Kryszewska & K. Leksowski (Eds.), *Healthcare Administration for Patient Safety and Engagement* (pp. 106–119). Hershey, PA: IGI Global. doi:10.4018/978-1-5225-3946-9.ch006

Rosiek, A., Leksowski, K., Goch, A., Rosiek-Kryszewska, A., & Leksowski, Ł. (2016). Medical Treatment and Difficult Ethical Decisions in Interdisciplinary Hospital Teams. In A. Rosiek & K. Leksowski (Eds.), *Organizational Culture and Ethics in Modern Medicine* (pp. 121–153). Hershey, PA: IGI Global. doi:10.4018/978-1-4666-9658-7.ch006

Rosiek, A., & Rosiek-Kryszewska, A. (2018). Managed Healthcare: Doctor Life Satisfaction and Its Impact on the Process of Communicating With the Patient. In A. Rosiek-Kryszewska & K. Leksowski (Eds.), *Healthcare Administration for Patient Safety and Engagement* (pp. 244–261). Hershey, PA: IGI Global. doi:10.4018/978-1-5225-3946-9.ch013

Rosiek-Kryszewska, A., Leksowski, Ł., Rosiek, A., Leksowski, K., & Goch, A. (2016). Clinical Communication in the Aspect of Development of New Technologies and E-Health in the Doctor-Patient Relationship. In A. Rosiek & K. Leksowski (Eds.), *Organizational Culture and Ethics in Modern Medicine* (pp. 18–51). Hershey, PA: IGI Global. doi:10.4018/978-1-4666-9658-7.ch002

Rosiek-Kryszewska, A., & Rosiek, A. (2018). The Involvement of the Patient and his Perspective Evaluation of the Quality of Healthcare. In A. Rosiek-Kryszewska & K. Leksowski (Eds.), *Healthcare Administration for Patient Safety and Engagement* (pp. 121–144). Hershey, PA: IGI Global. doi:10.4018/978-1-5225-3946-9.ch007

Rosiek-Kryszewska, A., & Rosiek, A. (2018). The Impact of Management and Leadership Roles in Building Competitive Healthcare Units. In A. Rosiek-Kryszewska & K. Leksowski (Eds.), *Healthcare Administration for Patient Safety and Engagement* (pp. 13–30). Hershey, PA: IGI Global. doi:10.4018/978-1-5225-3946-9.ch002

Roşu, S. M., Păvăloiu, I. B., Dragoi, G., Apostol, C. G., & Munteanu, D. (2016). Telemedicine Based on LMDS in the Urban/Metropolitan Area: A Romanian Case Study. In M. Cruz-Cunha, I. Miranda, R. Martinho, & R. Rijo (Eds.), *Encyclopedia of E-Health and Telemedicine* (pp. 96–109). Hershey, PA: IGI Global. doi:10.4018/978-1-4666-9978-6.ch009

Rouzbehani, K. (2017). Health Policy Implementation: Moving Beyond Its Barriers in United States. In N. Wickramasinghe (Ed.), *Handbook of Research on Healthcare Administration and Management* (pp. 541–552). Hershey, PA: IGI Global. doi:10.4018/978-1-5225-0920-2.ch032

Ruiz, I. M., Cohen, D. S., & Marco, Á. M. (2016). ISO/IEEE11073 Family of Standards: Trends and Applications on E-Health Monitoring. In M. Cruz-Cunha, I. Miranda, R. Martinho, & R. Rijo (Eds.), *Encyclopedia of E-Health and Telemedicine* (pp. 646–660). Hershey, PA: IGI Global. doi:10.4018/978-1-4666-9978-6.ch050

Sam, S. (2017). Mobile Phones and Expanding Human Capabilities in Plural Health Systems. In K. Moahi, K. Bwalya, & P. Sebina (Eds.), *Health Information Systems and the Advancement of Medical Practice in Developing Countries* (pp. 93–114). Hershey, PA: IGI Global. doi:10.4018/978-1-5225-2262-1.ch006

Sankaranarayanan, S., & Ganesan, S. (2016). Applications of Intelligent Agents in Health Sector-A Review. *International Journal of E-Health and Medical Communications*, *7*(1), 1–30. doi:10.4018/IJEHMC.2016010101

Santos-Trigo, M., Suaste, E., & Figuerola, P. (2018). Technology Design and Routes for Tool Appropriation in Medical Practices. In M. Khosrow-Pour, D.B.A. (Ed.), Encyclopedia of Information Science and Technology, Fourth Edition (pp. 3794-3804). Hershey, PA: IGI Global. doi:10.4018/978-1-5225-2255-3.ch329

Sarivougioukas, J., Vagelatos, A., Parsopoulos, K. E., & Lagaris, I. E. (2018). Home UbiHealth. In M. Khosrow-Pour, D.B.A. (Ed.), Encyclopedia of Information Science and Technology, Fourth Edition (pp. 7765-7774). Hershey, PA: IGI Global. doi:10.4018/978-1-5225-2255-3.ch675

Sarkar, B. K. (2017). Big Data and Healthcare Data: A Survey. *International Journal of Knowledge-Based Organizations*, *7*(4), 50–77. doi:10.4018/IJKBO.2017100104

Saxena, K., & Banodha, U. (2017). An Essence of the SOA on Healthcare. In R. Bhadoria, N. Chaudhari, G. Tomar, & S. Singh (Eds.), *Exploring Enterprise Service Bus in the Service-Oriented Architecture Paradigm* (pp. 283–304). Hershey, PA: IGI Global. doi:10.4018/978-1-5225-2157-0.ch018

Schmeida, M., & McNeal, R. (2016). Consulting Online Healthcare Information: E-Caregivers as Knowledgeable Decision Makers. *International Journal of Computers in Clinical Practice, 1*(1), 42–52. doi:10.4018/IJCCP.2016010104

Sen, K., & Ghosh, K. (2018). Incorporating Global Medical Knowledge to Solve Healthcare Problems: A Framework for a Crowdsourcing System. *International Journal of Healthcare Information Systems and Informatics, 13*(1), 1–14. doi:10.4018/IJHISI.2018010101

Shakdher, A., & Pandey, K. (2017). REDAlert+: Medical/Fire Emergency and Warning System using Android Devices. *International Journal of E-Health and Medical Communications, 8*(1), 37–51. doi:10.4018/IJEHMC.2017010103

Shekarian, E., Abdul-Rashid, S. H., & Olugu, E. U. (2017). An Integrated Fuzzy VIKOR Method for Performance Management in Healthcare. In M. Tavana, K. Szabat, & K. Puranam (Eds.), *Organizational Productivity and Performance Measurements Using Predictive Modeling and Analytics* (pp. 40–61). Hershey, PA: IGI Global. doi:10.4018/978-1-5225-0654-6.ch003

Shi, J., Erdem, E., & Liu, H. (2016). Expanding Role of Telephone Systems in Healthcare: Developments and Opportunities. In A. Dwivedi (Ed.), *Reshaping Medical Practice and Care with Health Information Systems* (pp. 87–131). Hershey, PA: IGI Global. doi:10.4018/978-1-4666-9870-3.ch004

Shijina, V., & John, S. J. (2017). Multiple Relations and its Application in Medical Diagnosis. *International Journal of Fuzzy System Applications, 6*(4), 47–62. doi:10.4018/IJFSA.2017100104

Shipley, N., & Chakraborty, J. (2018). Big Data and mHealth: Increasing the Usability of Healthcare Through the Customization of Pinterest – Literary Perspective. In J. Machado, A. Abelha, M. Santos, & F. Portela (Eds.), *Next-Generation Mobile and Pervasive Healthcare Solutions* (pp. 46–66). Hershey, PA: IGI Global. doi:10.4018/978-1-5225-2851-7.ch004

Singh, A., & Dutta, M. K. (2017). A Reversible Data Hiding Scheme for Efficient Management of Tele-Ophthalmological Data. *International Journal of E-Health and Medical Communications, 8*(3), 38–54. doi:10.4018/IJEHMC.2017070103

Sivaji, A., Radjo, H. K., Amin, M., & Abu Hashim, M. A. (2016). Design of a Hospital Interactive Wayfinding System: Designing for Malaysian Users. In N. Mohamed, T. Mantoro, M. Ayu, & M. Mahmud (Eds.), *Critical Socio-Technical Issues Surrounding Mobile Computing* (pp. 88–123). Hershey, PA: IGI Global. doi:10.4018/978-1-4666-9438-5.ch005

Skourti, P. K., & Pavlakis, A. (2017). The Second Victim Phenomenon: The Way Out. In M. Riga (Ed.), *Impact of Medical Errors and Malpractice on Health Economics, Quality, and Patient Safety* (pp. 197–222). Hershey, PA: IGI Global. doi:10.4018/978-1-5225-2337-6.ch008

Smith, C. R. (2018). Medical Students' Quest Towards the Long White Coat: Impact on Mental Health and Well-Being. In C. Smith (Ed.), *Exploring the Pressures of Medical Education From a Mental Health and Wellness Perspective* (pp. 1–42). Hershey, PA: IGI Global. doi:10.4018/978-1-5225-2811-1.ch001

Smith, S. I., & Dandignac, M. (2018). Perfectionism: Addressing Lofty Expectations in Medical School. In C. Smith (Ed.), *Exploring the Pressures of Medical Education From a Mental Health and Wellness Perspective* (pp. 68–91). Hershey, PA: IGI Global. doi:10.4018/978-1-5225-2811-1.ch003

Sobrinho, Á. A., Dias da Silva, L., Perkusich, A., Cunha, P., Pinheiro, M. E., & Melo de Medeiros, L. (2016). Towards Medical Systems to Aid the Detection and Treatment of Chronic Diseases. In D. Fotiadis (Ed.), *Handbook of Research on Trends in the Diagnosis and Treatment of Chronic Conditions* (pp. 50–69). Hershey, PA: IGI Global. doi:10.4018/978-1-4666-8828-5.ch003

Soczywko, J., & Rutkowska, D. (2018). The Patient/Provider Relationship in Emergency Medicine: Organization, Communication, and Understanding. In A. Rosiek-Kryszewska & K. Leksowski (Eds.), *Healthcare Administration for Patient Safety and Engagement* (pp. 74–105). Hershey, PA: IGI Global. doi:10.4018/978-1-5225-3946-9.ch005

Sołtysik-Piorunkiewicz, A., Furmankiewicz, M., & Ziuziański, P. (2016). Web Healthcare Applications in Poland: Trends, Standards, Barriers and Possibilities of Implementation and Usage of E-Health Systems. In I. Deliyannis, P. Kostagiolas, & C. Banou (Eds.), *Experimental Multimedia Systems for Interactivity and Strategic Innovation* (pp. 258–283). Hershey, PA: IGI Global. doi:10.4018/978-1-4666-8659-5.ch013

Soni, P. (2018). Implications of HIPAA and Subsequent Regulations on Information Technology. In M. Gupta, R. Sharman, J. Walp, & P. Mulgund (Eds.), *Information Technology Risk Management and Compliance in Modern Organizations* (pp. 71–98). Hershey, PA: IGI Global. doi:10.4018/978-1-5225-2604-9.ch004

Spinelli, R., & Benevolo, C. (2016). From Healthcare Services to E-Health Applications: A Delivery System-Based Taxonomy. In A. Dwivedi (Ed.), *Reshaping Medical Practice and Care with Health Information Systems* (pp. 205–245). Hershey, PA: IGI Global. doi:10.4018/978-1-4666-9870-3.ch007

Srivastava, A., & Aggarwal, A. K. (2018). Medical Image Fusion in Spatial and Transform Domain: A Comparative Analysis. In M. Anwar, A. Khosla, & R. Kapoor (Eds.), *Handbook of Research on Advanced Concepts in Real-Time Image and Video Processing* (pp. 281–300). Hershey, PA: IGI Global. doi:10.4018/978-1-5225-2848-7.ch011

Srivastava, S. K., & Roy, S. N. (2018). Recommendation System: A Potential Tool for Achieving Pervasive Health Care. In J. Machado, A. Abelha, M. Santos, & F. Portela (Eds.), *Next-Generation Mobile and Pervasive Healthcare Solutions* (pp. 111–127). Hershey, PA: IGI Global. doi:10.4018/978-1-5225-2851-7.ch008

Stancu, A. (2016). Correlations and Patterns of Food and Health Consumer Expenditure. In A. Jean-Vasile (Ed.), *Food Science, Production, and Engineering in Contemporary Economies* (pp. 44–101). Hershey, PA: IGI Global. doi:10.4018/978-1-5225-0341-5.ch003

Stanimirovic, D. (2017). Digitalization of Death Certification Model: Transformation Issues and Implementation Concerns. In S. Saeed, Y. Bamarouf, T. Ramayah, & S. Iqbal (Eds.), *Design Solutions for User-Centric Information Systems* (pp. 22–43). Hershey, PA: IGI Global. doi:10.4018/978-1-5225-1944-7.ch002

Stavros, A., Vavoulidis, E., & Nasioutziki, M. (2016). The Use of Mobile Health Applications for Quality Control and Accreditational Purposes in a Cytopathology Laboratory. In A. Moumtzoglou (Ed.), *M-Health Innovations for Patient-Centered Care* (pp. 262–283). Hershey, PA: IGI Global. doi:10.4018/978-1-4666-9861-1.ch013

Sukkird, V., & Shirahada, K. (2018). E-Health Service Model for Asian Developing Countries: A Case of Emergency Medical Service for Elderly People in Thailand. In M. Khosrow-Pour (Ed.), *Optimizing Current Practices in E-Services and Mobile Applications* (pp. 214–232). Hershey, PA: IGI Global. doi:10.4018/978-1-5225-5026-6.ch011

Sygit, B., & Wąsik, D. (2016). Patients' Rights and Medical Personnel Duties in the Field of Hospital Care. In A. Rosiek & K. Leksowski (Eds.), *Organizational Culture and Ethics in Modern Medicine* (pp. 282–297). Hershey, PA: IGI Global. doi:10.4018/978-1-4666-9658-7.ch012

Sygit, B., & Wąsik, D. (2016). The Idea of Human Rights in Conditions of Hospital Treatment. In A. Rosiek & K. Leksowski (Eds.), *Organizational Culture and Ethics in Modern Medicine* (pp. 236–254). Hershey, PA: IGI Global. doi:10.4018/978-1-4666-9658-7.ch010

Talbot, T. B. (2017). Making Lifelike Medical Games in the Age of Virtual Reality: An Update on "Playing Games with Biology" from 2013. In B. Dubbels (Ed.), *Transforming Gaming and Computer Simulation Technologies across Industries* (pp. 103–119). Hershey, PA: IGI Global. doi:10.4018/978-1-5225-1817-4.ch006

Tamposis, I., Pouliakis, A., Fezoulidis, I., & Karakitsos, P. (2016). Mobile Platforms Supporting Health Professionals: Need, Technical Requirements, and Applications. In A. Moumtzoglou (Ed.), *M-Health Innovations for Patient-Centered Care* (pp. 91–114). Hershey, PA: IGI Global. doi:10.4018/978-1-4666-9861-1.ch005

Tiago, M. T., Tiago, F., Amaral, F. E., & Silva, S. (2016). Healthy 3.0: Healthcare Digital Dimensions. In A. Dwivedi (Ed.), *Reshaping Medical Practice and Care with Health Information Systems* (pp. 287–322). Hershey, PA: IGI Global. doi:10.4018/978-1-4666-9870-3.ch010

Tripathy, B. (2016). Application of Rough Set Based Models in Medical Diagnosis. In S. Dash & B. Subudhi (Eds.), *Handbook of Research on Computational Intelligence Applications in Bioinformatics* (pp. 144–168). Hershey, PA: IGI Global. doi:10.4018/978-1-5225-0427-6.ch008

Turcu, C. E., & Turcu, C. O. (2017). Social Internet of Things in Healthcare: From Things to Social Things in Internet of Things. In C. Reis & M. Maximiano (Eds.), *Internet of Things and Advanced Application in Healthcare* (pp. 266–295). Hershey, PA: IGI Global. doi:10.4018/978-1-5225-1820-4.ch010

Unwin, D. W., Sanzogni, L., & Sandhu, K. (2017). Developing and Measuring the Business Case for Health Information Technology. In K. Moahi, K. Bwalya, & P. Sebina (Eds.), *Health Information Systems and the Advancement of Medical Practice in Developing Countries* (pp. 262–290). Hershey, PA: IGI Global. doi:10.4018/978-1-5225-2262-1.ch015

Urooj, S., & Singh, S. P. (2016). Wavelet Transform-Based Soft Computational Techniques and Applications in Medical Imaging. In P. Saxena, D. Singh, & M. Pant (Eds.), *Problem Solving and Uncertainty Modeling through Optimization and Soft Computing Applications* (pp. 339–363). Hershey, PA: IGI Global. doi:10.4018/978-1-4666-9885-7.ch016

Vasant, P. (2018). A General Medical Diagnosis System Formed by Artificial Neural Networks and Swarm Intelligence Techniques. In U. Kose, G. Guraksin, & O. Deperlioglu (Eds.), *Nature-Inspired Intelligent Techniques for Solving Biomedical Engineering Problems* (pp. 130–145). Hershey, PA: IGI Global. doi:10.4018/978-1-5225-4769-3.ch006

Waegemann, C. P. (2016). mHealth: History, Analysis, and Implementation. In A. Moumtzoglou (Ed.), M-Health Innovations for Patient-Centered Care (pp. 1-19). Hershey, PA: IGI Global. doi:10.4018/978-1-4666-9861-1.ch001

Watfa, M. K., Majeed, H., & Salahuddin, T. (2016). Computer Based E-Healthcare Clinical Systems: A Comprehensive Survey. *International Journal of Privacy and Health Information Management, 4*(1), 50–69. doi:10.4018/IJPHIM.2016010104

Wietholter, J. P., Coetzee, R., Nardella, B., Kincaid, S. E., & Slain, D. (2016). International Healthcare Experiences: Caring While Learning and Learning While Caring. In D. Velliaris & D. Coleman-George (Eds.), *Handbook of Research on Study Abroad Programs and Outbound Mobility* (pp. 470–496). Hershey, PA: IGI Global. doi:10.4018/978-1-5225-0169-5.ch019

Witzke, K., & Specht, O. (2017). M-Health Telemedicine and Telepresence in Oral and Maxillofacial Surgery: An Innovative Prehospital Healthcare Concept in Structurally Weak Areas. *International Journal of Reliable and Quality E-Healthcare, 6*(4), 37–48. doi:10.4018/IJRQEH.2017100105

Wójcik, A., & Chojnacki, M. (2016). Behavior and Ethical Problems in the Functioning of the Operating Theater (Case Study). In A. Rosiek & K. Leksowski (Eds.), *Organizational Culture and Ethics in Modern Medicine* (pp. 154–179). Hershey, PA: IGI Global. doi:10.4018/978-1-4666-9658-7.ch007

Wolk, K., & Marasek, K. P. (2016). Translation of Medical Texts using Neural Networks. *International Journal of Reliable and Quality E-Healthcare, 5*(4), 51–66. doi:10.4018/IJRQEH.2016100104

Wong, A. K., & Lo, M. F. (2018). Using Pervasive Computing for Sustainable Healthcare in an Aging Population. In B. Fong, A. Ng, & P. Yuen (Eds.), *Sustainable Health and Long-Term Care Solutions for an Aging Population* (pp. 187–202). Hershey, PA: IGI Global. doi:10.4018/978-1-5225-2633-9.ch010

Wu, W., Martin, B. C., & Ni, C. (2017). A Systematic Review of Competency-Based Education Effort in the Health Professions: Seeking Order Out of Chaos. In K. Rasmussen, P. Northrup, & R. Colson (Eds.), *Handbook of Research on Competency-Based Education in University Settings* (pp. 352–378). Hershey, PA: IGI Global. doi:10.4018/978-1-5225-0932-5.ch018

Yadav, N., Aliasgari, M., & Poellabauer, C. (2016). Mobile Healthcare in an Increasingly Connected Developing World. *International Journal of Privacy and Health Information Management*, *4*(2), 76–97. doi:10.4018/IJPHIM.2016070106

Yadav, S., Ekbal, A., Saha, S., Pathak, P. S., & Bhattacharyya, P. (2017). Patient Data De-Identification: A Conditional Random-Field-Based Supervised Approach. In S. Saha, A. Mandal, A. Narasimhamurthy, S. V, & S. Sangam (Eds.), Handbook of Research on Applied Cybernetics and Systems Science (pp. 234-253). Hershey, PA: IGI Global. doi:10.4018/978-1-5225-2498-4.ch011

Yu, B., Wijesekera, D., & Costa, P. C. (2017). Informed Consent in Healthcare: A Study Case of Genetic Services. In A. Moumtzoglou (Ed.), *Design, Development, and Integration of Reliable Electronic Healthcare Platforms* (pp. 211–242). Hershey, PA: IGI Global. doi:10.4018/978-1-5225-1724-5.ch013

Yu, B., Wijesekera, D., & Costa, P. C. (2017). Informed Consent in Electronic Medical Record Systems. In I. Management Association (Ed.), Healthcare Ethics and Training: Concepts, Methodologies, Tools, and Applications (pp. 1029-1049). Hershey, PA: IGI Global. doi:10.4018/978-1-5225-2237-9.ch049

Yu, M., Li, J., & Wang, W. (2017). Creative Life Experience among Students in Medical Education. In C. Zhou (Ed.), *Handbook of Research on Creative Problem-Solving Skill Development in Higher Education* (pp. 158–184). Hershey, PA: IGI Global. doi:10.4018/978-1-5225-0643-0.ch008

Zarour, K. (2017). Towards a Telehomecare in Algeria: Case of Diabetes Measurement and Remote Monitoring. *International Journal of E-Health and Medical Communications*, *8*(4), 61–80. doi:10.4018/IJEHMC.2017100104

Zavyalova, Y. V., Korzun, D. G., Meigal, A. Y., & Borodin, A. V. (2017). Towards the Development of Smart Spaces-Based Socio-Cyber-Medicine Systems. *International Journal of Embedded and Real-Time Communication Systems*, *8*(1), 45–63. doi:10.4018/IJERTCS.2017010104

Zeinali, A. A. (2018). Word Formation Study in Developing Naming Guidelines in the Translation of English Medical Terms Into Persian. In M. Khosrow-Pour, D.B.A. (Ed.), Encyclopedia of Information Science and Technology, Fourth Edition (pp. 5136-5147). Hershey, PA: IGI Global. doi:10.4018/978-1-5225-2255-3.ch446

Ziminski, T. B., Demurjian, S. A., Sanzi, E., & Agresta, T. (2016). Toward Integrating Healthcare Data and Systems: A Study of Architectural Alternatives. In T. Iyamu & A. Tatnall (Eds.), *Maximizing Healthcare Delivery and Management through Technology Integration* (pp. 270–304). Hershey, PA: IGI Global. doi:10.4018/978-1-4666-9446-0.ch016

Ziminski, T. B., Demurjian, S. A., Sanzi, E., Baihan, M., & Agresta, T. (2016). An Architectural Solution for Health Information Exchange. *International Journal of User-Driven Healthcare*, *6*(1), 65–103. doi:10.4018/IJUDH.2016010104

Zineldin, M., & Vasicheva, V. (2018). Reducing Medical Errors and Increasing Patient Safety: TRM and 5 Q's Approaches for Better Quality of Life. In *Technological Tools for Value-Based Sustainable Relationships in Health: Emerging Research and Opportunities* (pp. 87–115). Hershey, PA: IGI Global. doi:10.4018/978-1-5225-4091-5.ch005

About the Contributors

Sandeep Kautish is working as Professor & Dean-Academics with LBEF Campus, Kathmandu Nepal running in academic collaboration with Asia Pacific University of Technology & Innovation Malaysia. He is an academician by choice and backed with 17+ Years of work experience in academics including over 06 years in academic administration in various institutions of India and abroad. He has meritorious academic records throughout his academic career. He earned his bachelors, masters and doctorate degree in Computer Science on Intelligent Systems in Social Networks. He holds PG Diploma in Management also. His areas of research interest are Business Analytics, Machine Learning, Data Mining, and Information Systems. He has 40+ publications in his account and his research works has been published in reputed journals with high impact factor and SCI/SCIE/Scopus/WoS indexing. His research papers can be found at Computer Standards & Interfaces (SCI, Elsevier), Journal of Ambient Intelligence and Humanized Computing (SCIE, Springer). Also, he has authored/edited more than 07 books with reputed publishers i.e. Springer, Elsevier, Scrivener Wiley, De Gruyter, and IGI Global. He has been invited as Keynote Speaker at VIT Vellore (QS ranking with 801-1000) in 2019 for an International Virtual Conference. He filed one patent in the field of Solar Energy equipment using Artificial Intelligence in 2019. He is an editorial member/reviewer of various reputed SCI/SCIE journals i.e. Computer Communications (Elsevier), ACM Transactions on Internet Technology, Cluster Computing (Springer), Neural Computing and Applications (Springer), Journal of Intelligent Manufacturing (Springer), Multimedia Tools & Applications (Springer), Computational Intelligence (Wiley), Australasian Journal of Information Systems (AJIS, International Journal of Decision Support System Technology (IGI Global USA), International Journal of Image Mining (Inderscience). He has supervised one PhD in Computer Science as a co-supervisor at Bharathiar University Coimbatore. Presently two doctoral scholars are pursuing their PhD under his supervision in different application areas of Machine Learning. He is a recognized academician as Session Chair/PhD thesis examiner at various international universities of reputes i.e. University of Kufa,

University of Babylon, Polytechnic University of the Philippines (PUP), University of Madras, Anna University Chennai, Savitribai Phule Pune University, M.S. University, Tirunelveli, and various other Technical Universities.

Google Scholar - https://scholar.google.co.in/citations?user=O3mUpVQAAAAJ&hl=en
Linkedin Profile - https://www.linkedin.com/in/sandeep-k-40316b20/
ORCID Profile - https://orcid.org/0000-0001-5120-5741
More details about the academic profile can be found at www.sandeepkautish.com

* * *

Mohan Allam is a research scholar in the Department of Computer Science, Pondicherry University, Puducherry, India. He has been working as an Assistant Professor at Shri Vishnu Engineering College for Women, Bhimavaram. His research interests include Soft Computing and Image Processing.

Vinay Bhatia is a B.Tech, M.Tech, Ph.D, in Electronics and Communication Engineering. Currently he is serving as Professor and Head, Department of Electronics and Communication Engineering at Chandigarh Engineering College, CGC Landran, Punjab, INDIA. He has authored various research papers in various national/international conferences/journals. He is recipient of awards such as INDO-SL International award in the category of Best Head of Department, Academic Leader I2OR International Award 2020-21 etc. Currently he is working on routing and security issues pertaining to wireless networks. He is instrumental in development of Center of Excellence in ECE department at CGC, Landran in field of Drone technology and antennas of wireless communication. He has received a grant of from AICTE under MODROB scheme and travel grant from SERB, DST. He has been editor to various journals of international repute. His main research interests include wireless communication and its applications.

Jyoti Bhola has done her B. Tech. in Electronics and Communication Engineering from Kurukshetra University. She did her M. Tech. in Electronics and Communication Engineering, from Punjab Technical University, Jalandhar. She did her PhD from National Institute of Technology, Hamirpur in Electronics and Communication and currently working as Assistant Professor at Madanpalle Institute of Technology and Science, Andhra Pradesh, India. Her area of interest is Wireless Sensors Networks and Adhoc Networks.

Saksham Chaturvedi is a meticulous undergraduate pursuing Bachelor of Technology in Computer Science at Jaypee University of Information Technology, Wakhnaghat, Solan, Himachal Pradesh. His research interests include Artificial Intelligence, Brain-Computer Interface and developments in the field of Human-Computer Interaction.

S. B. Goyal had completed PhD in the Computer Science & Engineering in 2012 from India and served many institutions in many different academic and administrative positions. He is holding 19+ years experience at national and international level. He has peerless inquisitiveness and enthusiasm to get abreast with the latest development in the IT field. He has good command over Industry Revolution (IR) 4.0 technologies like Big-Data, Data Science, Artificial Intelligence & Blockchain, computer networking, deep learning etc. He is the first one to introduce IR 4.0 including Blockchain technology in the academic curriculum in Malaysian Universities. He had participated in many panel discussions on IR 4.0 technologies at academia as well as industry platforms. He is holding 19+ years' experience in academia at National & International level. He is serving as a reviewer or guest editors in many Journals published by Inderscience, IGI Global, Springer. He is contributing as a Co-Editor in many Scopus books. He had contributed in many Scopus/ SCI Journal/ conferences. Currently, Dr Goyal is associated as a Director, Faculty of Information Technology, City University, Malaysia.

Vishal Goyal, Professor, Department of Computer Science, Punjabi University Patiala, Punjab, with 20 years of Teaching and 3 years of Software Industry Experience, His research areas are NLP, Technology Development for Differently Abled People and Machine learning. Prof. Goyal is an Editor-in-Chief for an International journal – "Research Cell: An International Journal of Engineering Sciences". He is NAAC assessor and visited many Colleges for this purpose officially sent by NAAC. He is Co-Coordinator for "Center for Artificial Intelligence and Data Science". He is Coordinator for "Research Centre for technology Development for Differently Abled Persons" recently established at his University. He is Deputy Director of Centre for E-Learning and Teaching Excellence. He is an Associate Editor of SCI journal- TALLIP. He has developed many applications that are directly helping the society in making their lives better. He has been awarded Young Scientist Award in 2015 by Punjab Academy of Sciences, two times State award by Punjab Govt. He has into his credit ten copyrighted software, one trademark and two patents. He is currently guiding 08 Ph.D. students and 15 students have already been awarded doctorate degrees. He has guided about 120 M.Tech./M.Phil(CS) students for their major research projects. He has already completed projects worth 1 crore rupees and above funded by various Ministries of Govt. of India. He is recently been sanctioned project on Corpus development for Kashmiri, Urdu and Dogri worth 75 Lakh rupees approx. by Govt. of India Ministry. He has about 80 research publications in various journals of National and International repute, National and International Conferences. He has delivered about 100 keynote address, Inaugural addresses, invited talks in various conferences of National and International repute. He has also recorded 11 video lectures on DBMS at EMRC Patiala as part of their MHRD Project which are uploaded on CEC Website for open access. He was PI of MOOCs Programme on Cyber Laws available at Swayam Portal and this MOOCs programme has already been executed two times. He has into his credit six books published with well known International Publishers. He is Coordinator of NPTEL Local Chapter of Punjabi University Patiala. He has organized many conferences and workshops. He is regularly been interviewed by various TV Channels and Radio partners for their research on NLP and Technology development for Differently Abled Persons. He has been offered honorary position of IT Consultant at Maharaja Bhupinder Singh Punjab Sports University, Patiala. He is IT Subject Expert of Punjab School Education Board, Mohali. His detailed biodata can be seen at his website http://www.vishalpup.in/.

Vishal Jagota has done his B.E. in Mechanical Engineering from Maharishi Dayanand University, Rohtak. He did his M. Tech. in Mechanical Engineering & Machine Design, from Punjab Technical University, Jalandhar. He did his Ph.D. from National Institute of Technology, Hamirpur in Mechanical Engineering and currently working as Assistant Professor at Madanpalle Institute of Technology & Science, Andhra Pradesh, India. His area of interest are Material Characterization, Tribology, Heat Treatment of Steel, Statistical analysis and Simulation.

Malik Mustafa Mohammad Jawarneh is working at Gulf College, Muscat, Oman.

Rubal Jeet is working as Assistant Professor at Department of Computer Science Engineering Chandigarh Engineering College Landran, Punjab, India.

Nandhini M. has been working as an Associate Professor in the Department of Computer Science, Pondicherry University, Puducherry, India. She has completed her Ph.D. in the area of data mining. She has more than forty six publications in national and international journals and has presented twenty-four papers in international conferences of repute. She has published three books and two book chapters. She is a reviewer of SCI-indexed journals. She has delivered many invited talks at the national workshops and FDPs. Her research areas include Data mining, Artificial Intelligence, Software Engineering, Evolutionary Algorithms, and Combinatorial Problem Optimization.

Vinay Kumar Nassa belongs to Sonepat (Hr.). He did B.E(Electronics) from Nagpur University. He obtained two Postgraduate degrees M.C.A from M.D.U Rohtak (2004) & M.Tech (ECE) from P.T.U, Jalandhar in 2007. He also did PhD in Computer Engg. & ECE. He has blend of knowledge in both the fields and most of his experience is in teaching M.C.A & M. Tech. In addition to this he is a member of various professionals bodies like CSI, IEEE, ISTE & IANGE etc. He is in panel of revivers of many National & International Journals. He has 26 years of teaching and 5 years of industry. He had experience of establishing of new institutes and worked as Director/Principal of Various Institutions.

Shadab Pattekari is a director with thirteen years of experience working alongside the executive team of Indala Group of Institutions. Shadab specializes in administrative technology and is responsible for educating other employees on using progressive education systems. Shadab is a powerful force in the workplace and uses his positive attitude and tireless energy to encourage others to work hard and succeed. Shadab is inspired daily by his wife and their children's. In his free time, Shadab likes to learn new technologies.

Arun B. Prasad is Area Head, Humanities and Commerce at Institute of Law. He is Doctorate in the area of Health Economics. In a career spanning 14 years, he has taught in different branches such as Arts, Commerce, Management, Technology and Law. With rich experience in UG and PG level, he has been involved in curriculum development and academic administration. He is teaching courses related to Economics, Entrepreneurship and allied areas such as Micro/Macro Economics, Economic Development and Policy, Money and Capital Market. Presently, he is In-Charge of IQAC at Institute Level. He is the member of the following forums: 1. Gujarat Economics Association 2. Ahmedabad Management Association 3. National Editorial Board, Indian Journal of Law and Human Behavior, ISSN 2454-7107 (New Delhi) – Continuing 2019 4. Member, Center of Corporate Law Studies - Institute of Law, Nirma University.

Himayun Qureshi is an MTech from BITS Pilani in Embedded Systems. Patent holder for next generation Framework for Smart Building Monitoring using 6LoWPAN. Area of interest includes internet of things, machine learning, artificial intelligence, and deep learning. Main focus is teaching research in STEM.

Mohammad Shabaz has received his B.Tech in Information Technology and Telecommunication from Baba Ghulam Shah Badshah University and MTech, Ph.D from Chandigarh University, India. He is currently working as Assistant Professor at Chitkara University, India. He has published Research Papers in International Journals including Scopus Indexed and Web of Sciences.

Aman Sharma is currently working as Assistant Professor (SG) in the Department of Computer Science & Engineering at Jaypee University of Information Technology, Waknaghat, Solan, Himachal Pradesh. He has around 6.5 years of teaching and research experience. He has completed his Ph.D. thesis in Computer Science & Engineering Department from Thapar Institute of Engineering and Technology, Patiala, Punjab. He obtained his M.E. in Computer Science & Engineering from Thapar Institute of Engineering and Technology, Patiala, Punjab. He has obtained his B.Tech. in Computer Science & Engineering from R.B.I.E.B.T, Mohali, Punjab. He has been a rank holder throughout his studies. He has also obtained A.I.R-1800 in GATE 2013.

Tarun Singhal has done PhD in electronics and communication engineering from MDU, Rohatak. His area of specialisation is Nano Electronics. He has total teaching experience of 13 years.

Praveen Singla is working as Assistant Professor at CEC-CGC Landran.

Garima Verma has done a doctorate in Computer Science Engineering from DIT University in 2018. She is UGC Net Qualified in Computer Science, Gold Medalist in MTech, Computer Science and Engineering from Uttarakhand Technical University. She has over 17 yrs of industry and academic experience. She has 37 (WoS and Scopus) Research papers in various reputed peer-reviewed journals and presented a paper in various conferences of international repute. She has worked with CMC Ltd as a software developer and NIET Greater Noida as an Assistant Professor. Currently, she is working as an Assistant Professor at the School of Computing DIT University.

Luis Vives was born in Chiclayo, Peru, in 1984. He received the Bachelor of Engineering Systems Lord of Sipan University in 2006. is currently studying for a doctorate in engineering from the Pontifical Catholic University of Peru. He is currently a professor in the Computer Science Career at the Peruvian University of Applied Sciences. His areas of interest are Software Engineering and Computer Science. His research interests being Software quality, software architecture, machine learning, knowledge extraction based on the semantic web.

Index

CPSIA information can be obtained
at www.ICGtesting.com
Printed in the USA
BVHW091949160821
614571BV00003B/45